Injured . . . What Now?

Hans-Wilhelm Müller-Wohlfahrt
Hans Jürgen Montag

Hastings House Book Publishers
Norwalk, Connecticut
USA

**Injured ...What Now?
is dedicated to sports enthusiasts everywhere.**

Acknowledgments:
  Hastings House would like to extend special recognition to the following
  people for their enthusiasm, patience, curiosity, and good humor:
Edited by <u>Vallerie Huyghue</u> and <u>Rachel Borst</u>, Hastings House.
Copy edited by <u>Earl Steinbicker</u>, Hastings House.
Layout design by <u>Mark Salore</u>, Landmark Document Services.
<u>Shanti Coble, Translations</u>, for initial translation of the German manuscript.

Peter Leers, Hastings House, for final translation of the German manuscript.
Dr. Andreas Marx, for his assistance in supplying U.S. equivalents to the German medications.
Joseph Sheehan, Assistant Athletic Trainer for the NFL's Jacksonville Jaguars, who offered advice and recommended bandages and salves used by athletes in the U.S.
Ginny Hull, Hull Graphic Design, for her beautiful cover artwork.

While every effort has been made to insure accuracy, neither the author nor the publisher assumes legal responsibility for any consequences arising from the use of this book or the information it contains.

Distributed to the trade by National Book Network, Lanham, MD.
Copyright © 1999 by Hastings House Book Publishers.
Cover by Ginny Hull, Hull Graphic Design.
Photos by Michael Westermann, Munich and Holger Nagel, Kehl a.Rh., Germany.

ISBN: 0-8038-9442-2
Library of Congress Catalog Card Number
Printed in the United States of America
10 9 8 7 6 5 4 3 2 1

Publishers Note

Injured...What Now? introduces the American public to Dr. Müller-Wohlfahrt, international expert on sports injuries and therapeutic treatments. He is team doctor for the most outstanding soccer club in Germany — FC Bayern Munich. Highly regarded within the sports community, he also runs a sports medicine and orthopedics clinic in Munich and London.

Germany is the leading country in homeopathic medicine. Physicians there choose from a wide variety of alternative and homeopathic treatments without dangerous side effects. Injured...What Now? describes these products, which have been used by Germany's top athletes for decades. Now, at last, this information is available to the American public.

In the past 20 years, the U.S. has undergone a renaissance in Health awareness. People now realize there are many alternatives to standard medical practices. In almost every neighborhood there are health food stores which supply homeopathic remedies based on natural products. Dr. Müller-Wohlfahrt strongly advocates the use of these products.

This book does not provide guaranteed therapy for every kind of injury — we suggest you consult your doctor whenever an injury occurs. We also suggest that you obtain your doctor's advice on medication and treatment regarding your individual situation.

Peter Leers, Publisher
Hastings House Book Publishers
Norwalk, CT

Good health cannot be overestimated; health is the highest goal for a human being — who does not know this? When one feels well, hardly a thought is spent on it. However, when physical fitness is lost — for whatever reason — much time and money is required to regain it, if at all possible. Many sports enthusiasts — from children and teenagers at play, and adults who engage in sports as a weekend hobby, to the professional athlete — have had the frustrating experience of problems due to sports injuries.

Injured athletes are often found in doctors' waiting rooms, with follow-up visits continuing for several weeks or months. Sometimes their work as professional athletes suffers due to injury-related absences. This may result in considerable financial loss. They torture themselves in work-out rooms and fitness clubs, exercising repeatedly to restore their performance.

Prevention — that is the best medicine. In their book Injured... What Now?, Dr. Hans-Wilhelm Müller-Wohlfahrt and sports physiotherapist Hans Jürgen Montag offer valuable advice for avoiding injuries. Yet, if injuries do occur, these exceptional medical specialists explain precisely what to do in each special situation.

Their book is intended to be a ready-reference source for parents, coaches, youth, and adults in all varieties of sports. Physical education teachers, in particular, have profound responsibility; in critical situations they are first to be called upon to decide what to do. <u>Injured... What Now?</u> offers quick, effective emergency measures, depending upon the injury. It offers valuable assistance, not only to trainers, but also to amateur and professional athletes who suffer sports-related injuries. This book belongs in every sports bag

Yours,

Franz Beckenbauer
Former Cosmos Star

Racing With Time

Example One: At an NFL playoff game in 1996 an AFC player, who will soon receive the MVP Award — limps across the field towards his team's sideline. There, the team's physician and head coach are awaiting him. Within seconds, the injured football star receives the best medical care that is possible. A few days later he plays again, in spite of a torn muscle fiber.

First, diagnosis; then instant treatment. In the locker room, additional measures are taken. Top athletes receive around-the-clock services; these injured stars are truly provided with the best in medical care.

Daily training continues and winning the next game is the top priority. The injured player is cared for with the highest commitment of medical professionals, along with state-of-the-art equipment and the most expensive treatments. It is customary for the professional football player — as with top athletes of other sports — to receive optimal care. Trained experts are always there to help.

Most people, however, are untrained in handling common sports injuries. With the help of this book, you can learn to take action the moment an injury occurs...<u>when every minute counts!</u>

Example Two: The kids of the Youth League compete on a soccer field for the ball, goals, and points. All are laughing. The game is played fairly, but with youthful exuberance. Sports should be fun; it's all part of the game.

And then, the accident happens: two boys wrestle to the ground; one remains lying there, moaning with pain. His knee is swollen. His teammates stand by sympathetically. Even the players from the other side, parents and coaches, come rushing to the scene. Standing in a circle around the injured boy, the on-lookers want to help. Their body language expresses the helplessness they feel. Not even a first aid kit is in evidence beside the team's bench. The boy cries. Yet, he cannot get more than the comforting words of the coach; his mother and father can give no more than an encouraging pat at this moment. Such situations must come to an end on playing fields, gyms and in recreation areas; they should be remedied in all places where people practice sports. It is for this reason that this book has been written.

The injured boy in example two was lucky. His knee was only twisted. Although he was unable to complete the game, his tears were soon dried and his pain soon forgotten. Only a few days later, he was running about with his friends. The following weekend, there was another soccer game. The boy appeared in uniform and ready to play. But again, there was no first aid kit near the home team bench. Surely, nothing bad will happen...

Responsible trainers, coaches, and those who want to be of help in serious situations must insure that the lack of preparation is ended. This book addresses itself to these people. It contains many valuable tips about handling sports injuries of all kinds.

Many valuable insights have been written by two leaders in the field of sports-injury therapy: Dr. Hans-Wilhelm Müller-Wohlfahrt, team-physician of the FC Bayern of Munich and the German National Soccer Team; and his colleague Hans Jürgen Montag, former sports physiotherapist of the German Soccer Association and the German National Hockey team at five Olympic games. Their book belongs in every athlete's bag.

Naturally, this book is not guaranteed therapy for every kind of injury — we recommend that you consult a doctor or other licensed practitioner whenever an injury occurs. Injured... What

INTRODUCTION

<u>Now?</u> is designed as a reference book for the most common and persistent sports-related injuries.

"What to do?" How often this question is posed on the sidelines of soccer fields, on the perimeter of the running track, at swimming pools and gymnasiums for basketball, or handball — and elsewhere — can only be estimated. Now, through this book, everyone has the opportunity to acquire the fundamental qualifications for first aid in emergencies and minor injury situations which often result from athletic activity.

Not all athletes are as lucky as the boy at the soccer game. Of the millions who participate in sports, thousands deal with injuries ranging from minor wounds to major trauma. These injuries can cause permanent health problems, and also serious professional and financial consequences.

Aid given within the first few minutes often determines the gravity and duration of an injury. Correct first aid could prevent prolonged recuperation. Informed help is needed. The authors provide expert instruction in a useful, concise, and understandable form. Advice on prevention, practical tips for avoiding future errors, suggestions for correct warming-up and cooling-down, as well as a taping guide, are also contained in this book.

Part I: Injuries

CONTENTS

Part II: Inflammations

Part III: Practical Tips

Part IV: Tapes

Part V: First Aid Kit

Part VI: Appendix

METATARSAL CONTUSIONS
(injured arches of the feet)

Bruises are a common occurrence in sports, especially contact sports such as ice hockey, football, rugby, and soccer. They must not be taken lightly, as serious problems can arise from inattention.

In the area of the metatarsus (arch), extremely painful injuries may occur. Improper distribution of weight leads to additional deterioration, forming a vicious cycle.

Caution: With a metatarsal contusion, the bone surface, tendons, or joint capsular/ligament area can become injured. If, for instance, a soccer player lands on the arch of his opponent's foot, the alignment of the joints may change, or one or several bones of the foot may break.

Symptoms

Athletes experience pain and increased difficulty when placing weight on the foot. Usually there is excessive bruising, with swelling in the affected area. Frequently, impressions of the opponent's cleats are imprinted on the top of the foot after an encounter.

Causes

Bruises are caused by an impact from a hit, blow, or kick; especially in the various encounters between two soccer players.

First Aid

First, examine the foot for cuts or abrasions; disinfect them using, for example, Mercurochrome or peroxide. Subsequently, apply an antibiotic ointment.

If no skin is broken, cool the injured area with Mineral Ice, and wrap with an Ace bandage. In the case of a skin injury, make a "hot-ice" bandage: Place a sponge saturated with ice water beneath a wet Ace bandage (3-inch width) and fasten it with slight tension.

If, when standing upright, there is a stabbing pain or a grating sound — similar to the noise of forming a snowball — the foot must be immediately relieved of weight. There is a distinct possibility of a bone injury. In this case do not use pressure bandages! Avoid weight bearing; a trip to the doctor is in order.

If treatment is unavoidably delayed, the following is recommended until the patient can be treated by a doctor: Do not remove or cut off the shoe or sock; leave the shoe on as long as possible, even in the shower! The laced shoe acts as a temporary pressure bandage and halts any further swelling. Keep the foot elevated above the level of the heart and continue to cool it with ice water until medical care is rendered by a doctor.

For a minor contusion, it is advised to leave the shoe on for awhile. Pour ice water into the shoe through the laces or straps. The compression of the shoe (which fits tightly around the arch) and cold water will halt the bruising process. Pain usually diminishes after a few minutes.

If you fail to take a bruised arch seriously, and do not treat it (pressure bandage and ice water), the consequences may be severe. If the symptoms continue, sports activities must be discontinued. It is advised to leave the shoe on until a "hot-ice" pressure bandage has been prepared.

Follow-up Care

Measures to relieve swelling include positioning the foot above the level of the heart. Every 20 minutes you should apply a cold pack to the area. It is advisable to move the injured foot within pain-free limits; alternating periods of 7 seconds of tension with 10 seconds relaxation. Repeat the process 10 times.

If the skin is broken you can disinfect the area first using Betadine and then an antibiotic ointment. Spread the ointment on thickly and wrap with a sterile bandage. Do not cover the area with plastic; this occasionally leads to inflammation.

When the skin is not broken, apply ointment-bandages during the night, for example: Marco Sports Blue, Flexall; or use Luvos Mineral Earth.

Medications: Traumeel Tablets (2 tabs. 3x daily), Bromalin capsules (3 tabs. 2x daily), Wobenzym (10 tabs. 2x daily) or Traumeel drops. (Consult your doctor.)

FOOT DEFORMITIES

During training or competition, the feet withstand heavy strain in nearly every type of sport. Again and again they are stressed, especially if they vary from their ideal form (as in the common occurrence of variations involving the ankles or feet). This is the case for many athletes. When there is excessive strain on the feet, there is frequent stress around the toes, arches, instep, and ankle-joints. As the consequence of unusual positioning, the following results may occur: Muscle tension, joint-capsule and tendon irritation or inflammation, inflammation of bone surfaces, as well as problems with the joints of the knee, hip, groin and spine.

METATARSALGIA
(pain of the ball of the foot)

Persons with "spread-foot" frequently suffer from the formation of calluses and (oval shaped) corns under the toes (joints 2,3,4), and burning of the sole of the foot. The front of the foot is especially stressed. The "spread-foot" is the most frequent form of all incorrect foot positioning, usually caused by wearing shoes that are tight, high heeled or with cleats.

NEURALGIA
(nerve pain of the foot)

After constant stress, sometimes after arising in the morning, there is an acute, intense, burning pain of the bones of the ball of the foot. It can be caused by repetitive jumping or running exercises involving the front of the foot, especially on hard floors, as well as frequent changes of running surfaces. Stretching the tendon of the arch causes the foot to begin to flatten. In more serious cases, when pain occurs even during rest periods, sports activities must be discontinued and medical care sought.

First Aid

For acute complaints: Foot baths at about 82° F with bath salts (such as Dr. Scholl's Footbath or Batherapy from Para Labs), and a gentle foot massage will diminish pain and help promote relaxation.

For normal, daily stress: We recommend well-fitting shoes with good arch supports, or consulting a podiatrist (foot doctor) for orthotics (supports.)

During sports activities: Have special sports orthotics made. A tape bandage is also appropriate: Cut a piece of foam rubber (about 1x2 inches wide and a quarter-inch thick in the shape of a pear), and place on the ball of the foot. Wrap this with a 2-inch-wide Ace bandage and secure with several strips of tape (about 1-1/2 inches wide and 6-8 inches long) in such a way that the ends do not overlap at the back of the foot.

Best Advice: Step with the wrapped foot on the center of a 6-to-8-inch-long tape strip and wrap both ends around the foot. The elevation must not exert pressure on the toe joints! Under the flexible bandage, place 12 folds of gauze bandage of 2-1/2 inch width.

Medications: A copper-quartz-rosemary tincture can be applied to the skin, aspirin plus Vitamin C, or other drugs, can be taken for pain as directed by your doctor.

Follow-up Care/Prevention
1. Consistent use of orthopedic supports.
2. Well-fitting shoes with an innersole.
3. Foot exercises; a foot roller or shower shoes with a massaging innersole should be used. If possible a podiatrist should measure the distribution of the pressure on the foot.

FALLEN ARCHES

Fallen arches are usually an inherited condition. Frequent complaints are: Irritation of the tendons of the arch or muscle pain in the area of the toes. A pulling sensation which is usually not a sharp pain happens at irregular intervals in the calves. When the condition becomes worse, the discomfort is more frequent.

First Aid
Arch support inserts (foam or gel) for lifting the arch of the foot are helpful.

Follow-up Care
After making a slipper-cast of the sole of the foot, a podiatrist will provide an orthotic inlay; use special foot exercises to strengthen the muscles of the sole; and wear sport shoes with an innersole.

Important: If necessary, lose weight!

PES VALGUS (heel pain)

Problems in the area of the calcaneal (back) part of the foot include tension of the muscles of the calves; possible circulatory disturbances resulting from a steep angle of the heel-bone during running. The inner malleolus (inner ankle-bone) usually protrudes sharply.

First Aid / Prevention

This mal-position can be corrected through the use of a well-molded foot support and good shoe-lacing. Select shoes with a narrow heel guide (stable heel cap).

Recommendation: For teens and adults, use inserts to raise the heel up to 1-1/2 inches; exercise to strengthen the mid-sole. This decreases unnatural movement.

PERMANENTLY ELEVATED HEEL

This is genetically caused. The arch is shortened on both the inside and outside. This frequently causes a knob in the area of the Achilles tendon. Due to its high-positioned arch, no dynamic, fluid, heel-to-toe movement of the foot is possible. Conspicuous motion at the outer edge of the foot can be observed. The outer bands of the ankle joint are chronically over-stretched.

Additional complications may include: Twisting or spraining of the ankle, or difficulties with the Achilles tendons, muscle tension in the lower leg, pain in the instep and longitudinal arch, and heel spur. Irritation may extend from the area of the sole to the knee joints.

First Aid / Prevention

Correct the stance by providing orthotics or supports. Avoid long training on hard floors; use properly-fitted footwear.

FLATFEET

Flatfeet cause difficulty in raising the toes, especially after strenuous exercise. The foot turns outward for comfort. After jogging or running, irritation of the knee occurs due to twisting of the lower leg compared to the upper leg.

Swelling and sweaty feet may occur due to weakness of the foot muscles. Frequently, a weakness of connective tissue is the cause.

First Aid / Prevention

1. Correct-fitting footwear with orthotics provided by a podiatrist.
2. Exercise weak muscles in the foot or calf.
3. Walking and running practice with an experienced coach or trainer.
4. Careful attention to placing the foot straight forward.
5. A healthy lifestyle, omitting nicotine and other toxins.

Medications: Zinc supplements may be taken for 8 weeks (follow your doctor's directions), as well as amino acid supplements (e.g.: Glycine, Lysine, Proline), Vitamin A, Vitamin C, Vitamin E daily. (See your doctor for dosage.)

An accurate diagnosis regarding types of malpositioning of the foot can be obtained by seeing an orthopedic doctor or a podiatrist (who may use pressure distribution measurements and other specific tests).

Exercises for the prevention of foot injuries and strengthening of the foot musculature:

Example 1: Walk back and forth for 3 yards on the outer edge of the foot; repeat. Walk the same way on the inner edge of the foot, then the heels and the toes of the foot.

Example 2: Stand for 1 minute on each foot: 15 seconds each on the toes, heels, outer edge and inner edge of the foot. Repeat.

Tip 1:

Daily care of the feet should be routine for those in sports: Dry the feet thoroughly after the shower using a hair dryer, if available. Apply Vaseline or lotion when there is intense pressure due to hard floors, or after a prolonged break in training. Inspect your feet daily, especially the spaces between the toes and the around the nails. Trim your nails. Take foot baths. Massage your feet and do stretching exercises for the toes and arches.

Tip 2:

Have a mold of your feet made by a podiatrist in the afternoon after training, since the length and width of the feet change during the course of the day due to swelling. Also, purchase well-fitting athletic shoes after a thorough sports practice. When purchasing, always try on both left and right shoes and be sure to wear the socks or stockings that you expect to wear during sports.

INFLAMMATORY HEEL SPUR

The spur is a sharp, boney prominence of the heel. Inflammatory heel spur is an unpleasant, and frequently lengthy problem. The inflammation may become very painful, so that the affected person can no longer put weight on the heel or walk. Any sports activity is impossible. Often, the problem becomes chronic, so that inactivity can drag on for weeks or months if not appropriately treated.

Symptoms

People experience sharp heel pain during rolling-off or jumping movements and intense pain from weight-bearing. Pain of the heel is common in the morning. It is a specific, "point-shaped" pain when pressed with the fingertip.

Causes

Intensive, unvaried training routines (such as running only on asphalt) can lead to over-stress; as can games of tennis, badminton, squash, handball, or basketball on hard floors (concrete, asphalt). Repeated fast stops and constant jumping lead to problems of over-tiring of the feet.

There may be a gradual lowering of the longitudinal arch (which can lead to severe stress of the sole of the foot and subsequent inflammation).

Poorly shaped, worn-out shoes, a missing innersole, shoe heels that are too hard, ill-fitting supports, and some foot defects (such as flatfeet) may predispose the athlete to inflammatory heel spurs. In addition, gout (a disturbance of protein metabolism) is occasionally the cause of heel spurs.

First Aid

A physician or podiatrist can diagnose an inflammatory heel spur through the use of ultrasound and X-ray. A complete physical examination is recommended to rule out other causes of heel pain. An orthotic will provide relief of the inflammation. Additionally, shoes with firm heel guides are recommended.

Follow-up Care

Physical therapy is helpful when penetrating massage of the soles is included with stretching exercises of the calf and foot muscles. Medications may be injected or taken by mouth for pain.

The surgical removal of a heel spur is advised only in extreme cases, because the healing process can become very drawn-out.

Prevention

Provide good footwear; innersoles or inserts should be worn as a matter-of-course. Wear shoes with a strong heel guard. If pain is extreme, have an orthopedic doctor or podiatrist examine your feet and running style. For a precise diagnosis, training with video-taping is ideal. Have orthotics made for both sports and street-wear. After an initial visit with the doctor, have the orthotics checked regularly, and if necessary, adjusted. In recent years, the quality of flexible sport-shoe orthotics has improved enormously due to excellent materials and production methods. Prevention of recurrence can be insured by stretching the calf muscles, foot muscles, and stretching the tendons of the sole on an inclined plane.

Alternatively, perform the following exercise three times daily: Stand on a step of the staircase with the weight on the toes. Lower the heel as far as possible and hold for 7 seconds of stretching. Repeat the exercise 10 times, resting for 10 seconds between each set.

FORMATION OF BLISTERS

Regardless of preparation, blisters can happen quickly, especially on the feet. They represent a very painful injury to the skin. If not taken seriously they may become infected, particularly with "water" or "blood-blisters" which cause swelling of the lymph nodes (glands). Non-professional treatment is possible with small blisters, but larger ones need a doctor's care.

Symptoms

Blisters usually develop on heels, toes, fingers, or hands. At first, the affected skin holds up under uncommon stress from strong pressure or rubbing action. Then, an accumulation of fluid forms between the layers of the skin. A blister develops which, if large, can be very painful.

Causes

Poorly-fitting, tight, new, or not yet broken-in shoes, poorly-fitting socks or improperly wrapped bandages are often the cause of blisters. Foot blisters occur after pauses in training and from practicing on hard floors. Blisters on the hands and fingers result from improper grasping, wrong-sized handles or shoddy grip-bands on tennis rackets, and poorly-fitting gloves (such as those for golf). At first, the formation of blisters may not be noticeable. Once detected, careful attention must be paid.

First Aid

From the first indication of pain, sports activities must be interrupted. The over-stressed skin should be covered with a special blister bandage (for example, Compeed blister bandage) or moleskin. If the blister is already filled with fluid, cleanse the area with soap and disinfect it with peroxide. After washing your hands, pierce the blister carefully at the edge, using a thin, sterile needle, and disinfect once more, before covering the skin with a sterile bandage and ointment. Use the Compeed blister bandage and attach it in such a way that the affected area remains protected. Finally, fasten a protective, non-slip bandage around the dry skin. Through this process, the risk of tearing the blister open, with possible inflammation or infection, is avoided. Wet bandages must be replaced.

Follow-up Care

If a blister is extremely pressure-sensitive and painful, have it opened carefully. For blisters the size of a quarter or larger, minor emergency clinic care by a doctor is urgently advised. After draining the fluid from the blister, the pain is quickly relieved. In no case should you tear the blister or cut it! After proper opening and treatment, sports activities can usually be continued. For additional protection, cover the area with a clean bandage daily.

Important: Once the blister is opened do not cut or tear away the top layer of skin. Wait until the skin is dry and falls off by itself. It is the best protection for the underlying, newly-developing skin. Only shreds of skin should be cut off with scissors. During further sports activities, cover the damaged skin with an Ace bandage. Those who play racket sports or golf are advised to apply protection at the first twinge of pain from blisters on the fingers.

Prevention

Do not wear tight shoes. To relieve shoe pressure, spray the leather with a leather softener (Shoe-Eze is available from specialty shoe stores) and expand them overnight with shoe trees or newspaper rolls. New athletic shoes should be saturated with water and stretched until comfortably worn in. (During the wearing-in period, turn socks inside-out and lightly cover the toes, balls of the feet, and heels with Vaseline or lotion.)

Suggestions: Sports knee-highs or socks should be washed before they are worn for the first time in order to remove chemical deposits. Never wear socks that are too large or do not fit just right. Natural cotton socks and knee-highs are best without bothersome seams. Synthetic materials are not advisable. Also recommended are socks featuring reinforced cotton in the heels and toes. They are available from many sports shops.

NAIL BRUISES

This refers to any bleeding beneath the toenail or fingernail.

Symptoms

With bleeding under an injured nail, there occurs a red or blue discoloration of the nail bed. The affected area swells and causes increasing pain and pressure or throbbing underneath the nail.

Causes

Bruising of the fingers or toes from a hit, kick, or crushing injury may be the cause, however, even tight shoes or long fingernails can produce a nail hematoma.

First Aid

A sterile needle can be used to puncture a hole in the fingernail or toenail, and the blood released. This results in instantaneous relief of pain and pressure. Treatment need not be painful. Absolute sterility is a must! First, the feet (or hands) are carefully washed with warm water and soap, and disinfected with Bactine spray, Betadine or hydrogen peroxide. Gently scrub the injured toe or finger. To open the nail, use a sterile needle (available in most drugstores). Puncture the nail near the center of the bruise, using light pressure and a slight twist until blood flows out. Pain diminishes spontaneously.

Important: It is important to take care not to allow pieces of the nail to enter the puncture during opening. Afterward, the nail is doused with disinfectant and covered with a band-aid or flexible bandage covered with athletic tape. Attach the tape using gentle tension to avoid any further bleeding.

Caution: Due to the danger of infection, a minor emergency clinic doctor or other licensed medical professional should perform this treatment.

Follow-up Care

If a renewed throbbing is felt within the next 24 hours, the pressure should be relieved by the same procedure. The damaged nail should never be removed. Allow it to grow out naturally. It is the best protection for the nail bed. If the nail is removed, the nail bed becomes distorted and the new nail will be disfigured.

Prevention

No long toenails! Take care to use only correctly fitted footwear.

Hint: When possible, the purchase of shoes should take place in the afternoon and after training because the foot changes in length and width from exercise.

INJURIES OF THE ANKLE-JOINT

Ankle injuries are among the most common in sports. Regardless of whether you are a professional or weekend athlete, injuries of the ankle can happen anywhere and at anytime. Twisting the ankle or spraining it causes intense pain. The list of possible injuries is extensive: From a sprain caused by over-stretching ligaments and/or rupturing ligaments, to an injury of the cartilage or bone. Also possible are stress fractures or the rupture of a ligament/tendon union.

The correct procedure for any of these injuries is the urgent examination by a doctor to determine a diagnosis. Generally, this includes an X-ray. Avoid attempting treatment yourself. However, correct first aid of an ankle injury can have a very positive effect on subsequent treatment by the doctor (and the duration of the healing process).

Symptoms and Causes

Ankle injuries usually occur through the "buckling over" of the joint. This stresses the joint capsules (surrounding membrane) and the ligaments surrounding them beyond normal ranges, so that they become over-stretched. Either single or multiple ligaments may rupture (together with the capsule), depending on the mechanics of the accident. If there is no stabbing pain and no swelling, one can probably continue activity after a brief "hot ice" treatment. Afterward, a doctor should examine the firmness of the adjoining ligaments and follow-up the injury until healed. It is important to strengthen the muscles of the lower leg through exercise in order to stabilize the over-extended ligaments.

RUPTURE OF A LIGAMENT

An acute, intense, stabbing pain that occurs while turning the ankle inwards or outwards is usually a sign of a ruptured ligament. However, there is danger of underestimating this injury. Continuing to play or practice sports after acute pain can cause swelling of the injured area. It is even possible that there is almost no pain from a completely ruptured ligament soon after the injury. Soccer players often do not realize they have sustained a ruptured ligament — and the instability of foot that accompanies it — due to temporary compensation of well-trained musculature. They continue to play! If the muscle status is poor, the injured athlete who continues sports activities feels some instability of the foot.

The ankle tends to "twist" over again. At the first indication of pain, see your doctor!

SYNDESMOTIC RUPTURE
(ligament/tendon rupture)

A syndesmotic rupture happens between the shin-bone and the calf-bone. It may also occur with a ruptured ligament in the ankle, and be caused by an impact from kick or blow. It may also be caused by a mis-step. The rupture occurs according to a very particular mechanism: A forceful over-stretching of the front foot with simultaneous twisting of the heel toward the inside. Due to the absence of rapid, visible swelling — as would occur with the rupture of an outer ligament — the diagnosis is possible only through specific testing. The patient has severe pain during directional changes of the foot, especially from twisting outward over the rupture. It is impossible to exert pressure on the foot during jumps, sprints, quick starts or spurts. The transfer of force is no longer possible.

In this case, do not stress the foot. Use crutches and avoid weight-bearing as much as possible. Elevate the foot above the level of the heart with a "hot ice" pressure-bandage covering the painful area.

BONE INJURIES

Intense, unrelenting pain (often accompanied by nausea) may indicate a bone injury, such as splintering or fracture of the knuckles, calf, shin, or foot bones. Bone injuries are almost always accompanied by rapid and severe swelling. You must discontinue sports activities immediately. Do not put weight on an extremity until a doctor has provided treatment.

First Aid

Except in the case of mild sprains, all injuries in the area of the ankle generally require immediate cooling and compression. Injuries of the skin, such as abrasions, must be thoroughly disinfected (with Betadine or hydrogen peroxide) and covered with a plastic bandage. Finally, the patient has a "hot ice" pressure bandage applied. This is a sponge, saturated with ice water and held in place by a 3-inch-wide Ace bandage that has also been submerged in ice water. It is wrapped securely and firmly from the forefoot up to the middle of the lower leg. Position the foot high and wet the bandage from outside repeatedly with more ice water. Do not use ice-spray for this!

The sponge beneath the pressure bandage prevents additional swelling because it adapts itself to the contour of the joint. The pressure bandage, by itself, would allow swelling due to an absence of counter-pressure in some areas.

After 20 minutes, the pressure bandage must be removed for 3 to 5 minutes to allow blood to flow freely into the injured area. Until a doctor's exam, additional "hot ice" bandages are administered for a total of 3 hours.

Never use a pressure bandage if a fracture is suspected. (See chapter on "Fractures".)

If no surgical care or casting is required, use ointment-bandages after 3 hours of cooling. For skin injuries, non-irritating preparations (such as Traumeel or Neosporin ointment) are recommended.

If the skin is not broken, Marco Sport Blue or Cramergesic ointment should be generously applied to the injured area. A thin sponge, saturated with water, is laid upon it and wrapped with an Ace bandage. Keep the leg elevated above the center-of-gravity (abdomen).

Medications: The daily intake of, for example, Traumeel tabs,

Bromalin capsules, or Wobenzym, has proven beneficial in Europe. (See your doctor for correct dosage.)

Important: Leave the pressure bandage on during showering. Moreover, leave the bandage on at the doctor's office or clinic until the examination begins. The bandage may need to be loosened for an X-ray, and if waiting is prolonged, it should be reapplied until treated.

Caution: Because of the swelling, it is emphatically advised to refrain from the use of alcoholic beverages for the next 24 hours.

Follow-up Care

Only the doctor may decide about additional treatments and the resumption of training. It is very important for the injury to heal completely. Keep appointments for follow-up care. When the foot is free of pain, treatment should continue to help stabilize the condition. Otherwise, new injuries frequently occur from incomplete healing, especially in the area of the ankle. This may result in serious consequences, such as arthritis.

A physical therapy program — especially for the muscles of the lower leg, which support the damaged ligaments — must be initiated and supervised by a licensed physical therapist. Bad experiences have resulted from exercise programs supervised by amateurs. After initial instruction from a physical therapist, exercises using a therapy rubber band (check sporting goods stores) can be done at home. These exercises are inexpensive and effective.

After injuries to the ligaments, a podiatrist should provide a half-inch shoe elevation to the outer edge (to relieve the outer ligaments). This is to be worn for 4-6 weeks. Strained and over-stretching ligaments can be cured without any difficulty - if protection, good treatment and appropriate care are provided. These must be accompanied by supports or orthotics for both street and sports shoes.

Note: The muscles of the lower leg and foot are weakened from the use of a cast. That means that the foot tires much faster when training resumes. Depending upon the severity of the injury to the ligament, the foot can be given additional support through the use of Ace bandages, tape-bandages, or orthotics.

Tip: For training and competition, continue applying the support bandages for an additional 2-6 weeks. In the absence of pain, they should be worn until your stability is achieved again. However, use of the bandages should be gradually reduced over time. After recuperation, the bandages should be worn only during competition.

Important: At least once a year, an adjustment of the orthotics should be done because of possible material fatigue. For youths between 10 and 16 years, the inlays should be examined every 6 months.

Prevention

The athlete must work toward good, overall conditioning. The ideal is strengthening and firming the loosened ligaments and calf muscles through special exercises. The simplest form of prevention is to strengthen the foot muscles and the lower leg muscles by running barefoot on "natural ground" such as sand or grass. Writing the alphabet in the air with the toes will tone these muscles. Performing balancing exercises on a "Kreisel" (low-level balance beam) at the trainer's facilities or at the gym will provide excellent results.

In all types of sports, it is necessary to aim for good, over all conditioning. The greater the control of the foot through firm muscles, the less the danger of injury. To avoid injury, proper and well-maintained footwear is mandatory. Worn-out street and sports shoes with little or no stability in the soles allow "twisting" as do irregular and worn soles and supports. Check your footwear and repair or replace it, as necessary.

Note: During indoor sports such as basketball, volleyball, and handball, the ankle endures increased stress. Wear high-tops with padded soles. This applies especially to children who grow quickly and, therefore, have long limbs without correspondingly strong muscles.

IRRITATION OF THE ACHILLES TENDON

The Achilles tendon is the strongest tendon in the weakest area of the body. This oval shaped band serves to transfer power from the calf to the heel, and it is under immense pressure. During floor exercises, trampoline, and high-jumping, it supports 12-15 times the weight of the body. The Achilles tendon is constantly working because the legs are used from the morning until night. The Achilles tendon is positioned within a slide and, in contrast to other tendons, is not well protected, since it is not surrounded by muscles. Athletes who play football or soccer enter into one-on-one competition repeatedly. This is stressful on the body. Track and field athletes, gymnasts, and tennis players, place "explosive force" on the foot as it lands with pressure equal to many times the body's weight.

This area easily becomes irritated and, more rarely, develops an inflammation of the slide tissue (achillodynia), which envelops the tendon. In a worst-case scenario, the tendon may rupture under extreme stress or repeated injuries. This can only be treated by emergency surgery. In all cases of acute or chronic complaints, you must see your doctor.

Symptoms

When irritation of the Achilles tendon or its slide occurs, one experiences severe pain during movement, especially when "pushing-off" with the foot. The first steps in the morning are especially painful. Although the pain diminishes quickly with use, the symptoms recur after rest. The irritation is back again and the sliding resistance of the tendon canal is increased, as if by "sand in the gears." The tissue becomes inflamed, swells up, and there may be a slight reddening of the skin. The Achilles tendon becomes increasingly pressure-sensitive with extension. Sometimes, the tendon "creaks" when the feet are moved and makes a sound similar to the crunch of snow when a snowball is formed.

Athletes may not realize that there is a rupture of the Achilles tendon because they may still be able to run. They may feel as though some blunt object — like a stone — has hit the calf and may assume that it is merely a bruise.

A full rupture of the Achilles tendon is relatively rare and it usually occurs only after a prior injury. But, it can also happen while pushing a car, when the pressure exerted upon the tendon is extreme. During rupture, the pain is brief and dull. One hears a sound like the snap of a whip or a pistol shot, and can no longer "push-off" from the foot. However, it is still possible to limp. If the tendon ruptures, or has a 20% tear, surgery is necessary (in our opinion), at least for competitive athletes. In all cases of Achilles tendon pain consult your doctor for advice. Conservative treatments, such as casts only to decrease use, do not bring satisfactory results. After surgery, the tendon must be kept immobilized in a cast for several weeks. That is usually followed by 5 weeks of rehabilitation. After about 3 months, the patient is usually fit for sports activities.

Causes

A bruise caused by a kick (as in soccer) in the area of the Achilles tendon may result in the sliding-tissue of the tendon-canal becoming inflamed and swollen. Deposits and "cementing" can result in chronic problems. However, there may be many factors involved. Extreme stress in high-jumping and gymnastics, long-distance running, training on hard and unfamiliar surfaces, or a sudden change of the training surface from the gym into the open, or vice versa, as well as a loss of tone to shortened calf muscles can cause an irritation of the Achilles tendon.

Improper footwear, or chronic pressure by shoe components on the tendon, can contribute to an irritation. Moreover, foot deformities (e.g. a high arch) or an abnormal structure of the legs (e.g. "bowleg" or "knock-knee") may contribute. Even athletes who have back problems are more prone to irritation of the Achilles tendon. Gout and high cholesterol levels can lead to deposits in the area of the Achilles tendon. These cause irritation. Finally, general inflammatory processes must be taken into account, as well as inflammation of teeth or tonsils.

First Aid

After a blow or a hit on the Achilles tendon, it is advisable to immediately relieve or minimize both the swelling and inflammation that occur. A "hot ice" treatment with a sponge that is saturated with ice water and an Ace bandage should be immediately placed on the injured limb for 15 to 20 minutes. After a 4-5 minute interval, this process may be repeated 3 or 4 times. The bandage must be constantly soaked by pouring ice water on it at intervals. If necessary, the foot can be submerged in cold water (such as a bucket filled with ice-water). Do not place ice directly on the skin. Ice decreases circulation and, with it, the flow of oxygen to the already poorly oxygenated Achilles tendon. This will slow the healing process.

For 8 hours after the injury, apply a cooling ointment (such as Marco Sport Blue). Spread the ointment generously over the affected area, then place a wet gauze compress over it. Loosely wrap the Achilles tendon. Or, cut a piece of towel to the needed size, dampen with water, and spread on the ointment with a spatula. Lay this ointment compress on the Achilles tendon and wrap it. The tendon is stabilized and soothed.

For acute or chronic irritations, see a doctor.

Medications: Until the pain diminishes take Bromalin (2 tabs. 3X daily), or Wobenzym, Magnesium supplements and Traumeel tablets. (Consult your doctor for dosage.)

Follow-up Care

For the next 2-3 days, apply (mornings and evenings for 20-30 minutes per application) cold wraps with arnica tincture solution from Jurlique (2 Tbs. per pint of ice water). Leave the preparation in place until no further coldness is perceived. Meanwhile, repeatedly dampen the dressing with cold arnica tincture solution. At night, it is best to apply a healing earth pack (such as Luvos Mineral Earth), mixed with an arnica solution — which has been cooled in the refrigerator for several hours. These regulate heat in the injured area. Warmth is counter-productive to the healing process. During the day, an anti-inflammatory (for example, arnica tincture or Arnica SI ointment), should be applied to the injured area.

In addition, we recommend:
1. Stretches on an inclined plane for muscle relaxation.
2. Massage of the calves, upper legs and thigh muscles.

3. Foot baths with hydrotherapy (cool whirlpool for 20-30 minutes).
4. Examination by an experienced physical therapist or trainer.
5. Orthotics or insoles for sports and street shoes.

In acute cases, a gel-pad for a heel spur (such as Viskoheel) has proven effective for 2 or 3 days; it lifts the heel by about a half-inch, and tension on the tendon is decreased. The wedge should not be used for longer than 3 days, because the tendon must become re-adapted to normal stress. If there is pain, avoid stretching the Achilles tendon by jogging or training on the first few days after an injury. Replace these with other, less demanding training activities such as: Aqua jogging (which does not stress the foot), swimming, or bicycling without using the toes for pedaling. Exercise under the guidance of a knowledgeable trainer or physical therapist.

The full capacity of the Achilles tendon is usually regained through regular stretching exercises (see "Warming-Up"). Stand barefoot on the floor, slowly assuming a squatting posture until tension is felt in the calf (for 10 seconds). Or, step forward with the "good" foot while keeping weight on the injured leg behind (keep the knee joint straight). Shift your weight slowly to the "good" leg, while moving the whole body forward, until tension is again felt in the calf of the injured leg.

Important: The heels must remain on the floor. Perform this exercise daily; 10 repetitions within the pain-free zone.

Stretching on an inclined plane (done with the help of boards and telephone books) is also effective. Stand with both feet on a 4-to-5-foot-long board, at an inclination of 25-30°, with the heels placed lower than the front of the foot. Lean forward for up to 15 minutes. Then, stand for 5 minutes while facing opposite direction to relax the muscles. When no more pain occurs, gradually resume light training. After each period of exercise, cool the Achilles tendon with "hot ice" and a cooling ointment bandage (for example, Marco Sport Blue).

Train as little as possible on hard ground or Astro Turf. This turf has a hard sub-flooring that reverberates impact during running.

For athletes with Achilles tendon problems, training on soft, sandy ground is not advised. The heel sinks into the sand and the ground yields upon impact, so that the forefoot slips backward. This creates considerably greater stress on the tendon. Train on grass or cushioned track surfaces instead.

Prevention

Athletes with Achilles problems should avoid playing in cleats whenever possible.

Protect the Achilles tendon from kicks by wearing special calf guards with Achilles tendon protection during training and competition.

Wear shoes with maximum heel cushioning and proper fit. The heel needs an accurate guide and a firm hold. The heel-cap should be firmly connected to the sole and not reach too high, so that it does not press into the "slide-tissue" or the tendon.

When there is chronic irritation, have a shoemaker cover the heel of the insole with leather, allowing it to breathe. Otherwise, sweat on the heel is not absorbed and may become another factor for irritation. If there is weakness in the muscles of the lower leg, perform strengthening exercises to improve the condition. If the foot condition worsens, from foot deformities or swelling in the area of the ankle or sole, consult a physical therapist or podiatrist to promote healing through manual therapy. Foot supports, prepared by a prosthetics expert, are mandatory.

> **Tip:** For sports, 100% synthetic socks should be avoided. It is better to wear cotton which does not stiffen during washing. Wearing synthetic stockings and knee-highs can cause chafing, especially when there are Achilles tendon problems.

PERIOSTITIS (shin-splints)

Periostitis of the tibia (inflammation of the fibrous membrane along the bone's surface) is among the most painful of sports injuries, and can make practice for training or competition impossible.

It occurs most often in the lower-to-middle third of the inner side of the shinbone, and it develops from excess stress of the lower leg muscles, or after wearing ill-fitting footwear or supports. The deep calf muscles frequently cramp and cause "charley-horses".

When walking causes pain, training should be completely avoided.

Symptoms

The athlete may experience intense pain in the front and inside edges of the shin, usually during or after a quick start, running, or jumping. Pain in this area is typical when getting up in the morning. Walking on tiptoes is nearly impossible. Other symptoms include: Sharp pain from pressure, sometimes pain on touching, and noticeable swelling. Even pressure lightly applied with the finger on the affected area leaves a lasting depression, as do socks or knee-highs with elastic threads.

With acute inflammation, the patient can no longer wear stockings, knee-highs or shin guards because merely touching the area is painful. The deep muscles of the calf are also sensitive to pressure.

Causes

Shin-splints can have traumatic causes (kick or blow), but can develop due to overexertion, incorrect running style, and from footwear or supports that do not fit or were not well made. Over-stressed lower calf muscles and shin-splints develop from an unvaried and over-intensive training routine (such as performing repetitive stretches on an inclined surface). The new athlete who undergoes excessive training on hard ground (asphalt, Astro Turf, concrete) or uses inadequately padded sports shoes may develop problems.

First Aid

Use a loosely wrapped Ace bandage with "hot ice" and arnica tincture (2 Tbs. of arnica blended into 1 pint of ice water); saturate a sponge with it and loosely wrap the affected area. You can also prepare crushed ice in a knee-high (see "Practical Tips"), shape it around the injury, and wrap it with a wet towel. Place the pack around the elevated lower leg, using a short Ace bandage, and let it cool for 20 minutes. Repeat this therapy 3 or 4 times during the first 24 hours. Afterward, cover with ointment and bandages, such as Marco Sport Blue, or X-Cell-R-Aid salve. At night, a poultice with Luvos mineral earth pack (cooled in the refrigerator), an arnica-pack (for application, see "Practical Tips") or an ointment-bandage are recommended.

Medications: Recommended treatment depends on symptoms and includes the following: Traumeel tablets, Bromalin capsules or Wobenzym over a period of 10-14 days. (Consult your doctor for dosage and directions.)

Follow-up Care

Place an Ace bandage, which has been saturated in ice water

("hot ice") on the leg. Starting at the toes, continue over the ankle and up to the hollow of the knee. Support the foot comfortably so that it is above the level of the heart.

Follow-up exercises: Lie on the floor and place the injured foot on a chair. The exercise consists in pulling the toes toward the body. Hold this position for 7 seconds, and rest for 10 seconds. Repeat the exercise 10 times, followed by a two-minute pause. A total of 5 series "reps" are recommended. Following this, rub the foot, lower leg, knee and lower thigh with rubbing alcohol. Use a "smoothing" motion with both hands in the direction of the heart. For the next 3 or 4 days, you should apply a loose pressure bandage. Use a piece of foam saturated with Betadine. Apply to the injured area and wrap with a slightly-dampened Ace bandage that is three-quarters of an inch wide and cool from being refrigerated. Only slight tension is used for this wrap.

Providing the best possible shoes and supports helps with the healing process. The shoes should have a firm heel-cap and the insoles should be well-padded but not too soft. For additional support, place a layer of moleskin on the heel of the insole.

Prevention

1. Wearing shin-guards is mandatory for football, soccer, field and ice-hockey players.
2. Regular stretching exercises of the leg muscles, especially the calf muscles should be done consistently (see "Practical Tips".)
3. Train and play only on soft surfaces.
4. Use spikes sparingly. Field athletes should train only with sneakers; spikes should be worn only during competition.
5. Frequent running around curved surfaces should be avoided.
6. Avoid abrupt changes of ground, such as football

training on the lawn, followed by jogging practice on an asphalt track. (The muscles of well-trained athletes are so responsive and conditioned that — being sensitive to the abrupt change of foundation — they react with tension, which promotes the development of a periostitis of the shin-bone.)

Tip: Proceed cautiously with changes of training areas and shoes. Use alternating warm and cold baths to relieve stress from intensive, repetitive training. Submerge the lower legs to the knees in warm water (about 100 º F, ca. 36-38º C) for 2 minutes; afterward, submerge them in cold water for 15 seconds. Repeat 5-6 times. (Batherapy can be added to the warm water as a bath salt.)

Change the jogging style: After symptoms have diminished, check the athlete's running style in the mirror or by video recording; then have it analyzed by your trainer or physical therapist.

Rule: During all activities, refrain from turning the toes inward or outward ("pigeon-toed" or "duck walking"). Place the foot so that the toes point straight forward. Otherwise, the footsteps are "jolts" rather than spring-like. This needlessly stresses the muscles and joints, and disturbs their functioning. Moreover, the foot becomes fatigued and loses momentum.

Athletes who have a high instep (pes cavus) are especially vulnerable. If there are repeatedly, persistent problems — see your doctor! A specialist has to determine whether the cause for the complaint lies in the shin-bone itself (e.g., the possibility of a fatigue-fracture), or in the area of the lower back.

BRUISING OF THE SHIN-BONE (Tibia)

If the athlete has previously received an extremely painful kick in the shin, the pain is intense in the beginning, but diminishes quickly to a tolerable level. Yet, if it does not get treated, within minutes there is often a plum-sized swelling at that location. Without professional treatment, the result may be a serious problem, namely, periostitis (an inflammation of the bone covering). A thorough examination may reveal bleeding beneath the skin, or even a break in the skin.

Symptoms/Causes

In the beginning, there is severe local pain after a kick or blow. A bruise of the shin signifies an injury to the periosteum (the outer layer of the bone), because this bone has little soft covering. Bleeding in the tissues leads to pain from pressure. It can be easily treated. However, bleeding between bone and periosteum causes intense pain from stretching and pressure. There is pain to the touch.

First Aid

Cool with "hot ice" or "ice-slush" (see "Practical Tips") and apply an Ace bandage immediately. With an open wound, disinfect it first with Betadine or peroxide.

Follow-up Care

Rarely does a bruise force a game to end early. Because of the pain, the injured player needs to decide whether to continue or not. It is important to provide appropriate after-care with "hot ice" and a pressure bandage. Follow with ointment and bandages using Marco Sport Blue. At night, prepare a Luvos Mineral Earth with Arnica Gel Pack (see "Practical Tips"). For a skin injury, make an ointment-bandage using Traumeel ointment.

Medications: Bromalin capsules or Wobenzym and Traumeel drops. (See your doctor for advice and dosage.)

Prevention

Football, soccer, hockey players, etc., should never play without shin guards.

NOTES

All forms of Traumeel are available from:
Heel Inc.
1-800-621-7644

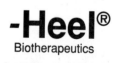
-**Heel**®
Biotherapeutics

INJURIES OF THE KNEE-JOINT

No other joint in the body undergoes more stress than the knee. It endures immense stress due to pressure, and it must transmit enormous amounts of energy. Amateur, as well as professional, athletes are vulnerable to knee injuries from sudden impact. Knee injuries have increased in almost every sport, with serious injuries (such as ruptured ligaments) occurring most frequently in football and skiing.

The knee is a complicated joint which can perform rolling, sliding, and rotating movements simultaneously. The possibilities of injuries are correspondingly complex. The internal and external ligaments may be involved, as well as the cruciate ligaments, the interior and exterior menisci (a crescent-shaped fibrous structure of the knee), the joint capsule, the articular cartilage (the covering which forms a joint), the patella (knee cap), or the patellar tendon. For any knee-joint injury, visit a doctor as soon as possible.

Symptoms

Depending on the type of injury, intense pain occurs in the areas of the interior joint, ligament, hollow of the knee (fossa), or the knee-cap.

The joint may feel "locked" or unstable. Frequently, swelling follows an increasing, sometimes overwhelming, feeling of pressure. Even when the pain diminishes, one should never underestimate any knee injury. Beware of having a false sense of security that nothing serious has happened. Always see your doctor.

Causes

Physical limitations are frequently the cause of knee injuries, especially in the case of amateurs. Many "weekend warriors" over-estimate their strength and are at greater risk than well-trained "pros". The danger of injury rises as fatigue increases. If the muscles fail to perform as needed, the ligaments (by themselves) are unable to keep the joint stable; it is possible for a cruciate ligament to rupture during a strenuous run without any external impact.

In our evaluation, the increase of knee injuries is the result of excessive demands on the athlete, especially in professional sports. In skiing, many knee injuries result from inflexible ski boots, which produce violent impact to the leg and traumatize the knee. In addition, further injury results from insufficiently-healed knee injuries.

First Aid

Never bend or stretch the knee-joint against resistance! Place the injured knee in a pain-free position (with a slight bend if possible). Elevate it above the level of the heart. Immediately visit a doctor who will make a diagnosis and give additional treatment.

If the visit to the doctor is delayed, cool the area using "hot ice" or "ice-slush."

Wrap with an Ace bandage (lined with an ice-water-saturated foam or sponge), under light pressure. The bandage should be applied over a large area — from the center of the lower leg (crus), to the center of the thigh. It is important to completely cover the knee-joint and to allow steady cooling of the entire joint. Do not force dramatic changes in skin temperature. A sustained, even cooling is the goal.

Important: Do not wrap the bandage too tightly, or "tie off" the joint; swelling may develop in the area of the crus. Do not cover the bandage with plastic wrap; it will prevent ventilation.

After 3 continuous hours of cooling, wrap the knee with ointment and bandages. In knee injuries with skin damage (such as abrasion or tears), the skin must be treated first to avoid infection. Place one of the following antiseptics on the open wound: Betadine, peroxide or Bactine. If none is available, rinse the wound with fresh, clear water (using a gentle flow) before wrapping with an antibiotic ointment-covered bandage.

Caution: Never rub a wound with a damp cloth or cotton swab. Never cover it with plastic wrap.

Follow-up Care

After cooling the joint, wrap with ointment and bandages (for example: Marco Sport Red, Traumeel ointment or Cramergesic). Spread the ointment (about a quarter-inch thick) with a spatula or tongue depressor directly on the injured joint, and cover with a dampened gauze bandage. Wrap gently with a pressure dressing. You may also cut a piece of absorbent cotton or rolled gauze to the desired size, wet the cloth with water and spread the ointment on it with a tongue depressor or spatula. Place it on the injured area and wrap with a flexible bandage. This should be replaced every 8 hours.

Medications: Pain-killers should be avoided prior to a doctor's examination. The patient's precise description of pain helps to establish a diagnosis. Later, the intake of anti-inflammatory drugs, such as Traumeel tablets and Bromalin capsules, follows. (Consult your doctor for advice and dosage.)

PLASTER CAST

Even though the indications for a plaster cast have diminished — due to the development of excellent synthetic materials — we do consider a cast appropriate for some cases such as an interior ligament rupture of the knee, or rupture above the talus (one of the bones of the heel), etc. A minimum of 10-14 days of absolute immobilization is essential for the injured ligament to heal in a useable position.

Follow-up Treatment/Rehabilitation

All knee injuries must be treated meticulously. We advise against attempted at-home treatment by unlicensed personnel. Rehabilitation and training should be guided and supervised by a doctor and an experienced physical therapist.

When the injured knee is free from irritation, pain during movement, or swelling, this does not indicate complete rehabilitation. Care must be taken to re-develop supporting muscles. This may be accomplished through supervised training. When the size difference between the weaker and the healthier upper thigh muscles amounts to no more than a quarter-inch, the rehabilitation is nearly complete. Permission for limited running can be given. However, one may wish to start with aqua-jogging and stationary bicycle training. After the rehabilitative exercises, we recommend the use of "hot ice" treatments which should also be applied whenever there is the slightest suspicion of over-use.

If pain returns, a doctor should be consulted. Pain is the natural warning signal of the body. The criteria for the resumption of training or competitive games is a totally pain-free knee.

Important: Knee bandages should not be worn longer than is absolutely necessary. If the sensation of strength and stability of the joint has been fully restored, discontinue support devices.

MUSCLE ATROPHY

Through isometric exercise one can limit muscular atrophy even when the injured leg is immobilized by a cast: Tense the upper thigh for about 7 seconds, then relax for 10 seconds. Repeat until the muscles tire. Pause for 2 minutes, then repeat the series.

Formerly, a muscle would lose one-and-a-half inches or more in circumference during 6 weeks in a cast. Now, the loss is merely three-quarters of an inch, due to accelerated therapy (14 days in the cast, then adjustable angular splints or Ace bandages for 4 weeks).

EFFUSIONS (swelling)

In case the knee-joint swells during the rehabilitation phase, reduce the intensity of stress. Elevate the knee and apply "hot-ice" bandages. Perform range-of-motion exercises in the pain-free-zone to cool off the joint. By cooling from the outside, the fluid moving within the joint is also cooled. Through range-of-motion exercises, the fluid spreads, cooling and calming the membranes within the joint.

[Also suggested: Cold packs (e.g. with a 40° F Luvos Mineral Earth Pack/arnica tincture mix).

During the day, ointment-bandages using Marco Sport Blue or X-Cell-R-Aid are recommended.]

Note: When there is a noticeable increase in swelling of the joint, with a simultaneous increase in pressure and heat development (usually a sign of inflammation): A doctor must be consulted. Swelling without much heat points to a mechanically caused reaction.

Prevention

The athletes' care of their own bodies is important. The body will forgive the mistreatment of youth, but through the years it takes revenge for irresponsible treatment. Tendencies toward injuries arise, especially of the muscles. Make time for maintenance of muscle tone and flexibility, as well as the training of weak areas. Pay attention to the conditions under which you train. Slowly recover ground lost through missed training and rest sufficiently after exercising in order to diminish the risk of injury.

Also: Carefully exercise the muscle groups that are important for joint stabilization. In the case of loose inner knee ligaments, strengthen the mid-thigh muscles. With a loose outer knee ligament, work to improve the outer-thigh muscles. (Consult a licensed trainer or physical therapist for instruction.)

Always include a 10-15 minute warming and stretching program before beginning any sports activity. (See "Practical Tips".)

This also applies to recreational athletes like skiers and hikers who must prepare their muscles and joints sufficiently before weekend outings.

Hint: Special muscle training should not take place on the day before a competitive game.

ARTHROSIS (joint degeneration)

Some older athletes experience increased movement-connected pain in the knees. Years of training and competition have left their mark. Additional damage may occur, usually in the cartilage. That is frequently the beginning of the development of joint degeneration.

Helpful: To strengthen upper thigh muscles: Bicycle (20 minutes), climb a hill, or exercise at a slight incline on the treadmill for 20 minutes.

Correction for mild "bowlegs" or "knock-knees": Use quarter-inch insoles for "knock-knees"; raise the outer edge by a half-inch for "bowlegs". Wear padded insoles, soft-soled or air-soled shoes, (Easy-Spirit, Nike, Dr. Martens, among others).

Medicinal Supplements: Gelatin, vitamins A, C, E, Zinc and Magnesium supplements. (Consult your doctor for advice and recommended dosage.)

PATELLAR LUXATION
(dislocated knee-cap)

When the knee-cap pops out of position the patient acts surprised because of the unusual appearance of the injury. They may have the impression that the entire knee is seriously injured. However, the knee-cap frequently pops back into position spontaneously. Because of the possible serious consequences of rupture or contusion of the joint-capsule or cartilage, immediate examination by a doctor is strongly advised.

Symptoms

The patient has intense pain from the knee. It immediately stiffens. The outline and form of the knee-joint changes. The patella "pokes out" palpably and visibly beside the knee-joint.

Causes

Violent side-impact may cause the patella to shift. This is usually caused by a fall or a mis-step taken with a stretched knee-joint and loose upper thigh muscles. However, a dislocation can also occur spontaneously, if the knee-cap is located in an unusual position: e.g. when the patella is too small, or lies too high above its gliding track on the upper thigh bone, or there is a deficient guide through the gliding track.

First Aid

If the knee-cap spontaneously returns to its track, discontinue all sports activities and visit a doctor. Keep the knee in a straight position — do not try to bend it. Cool the knee with "hot-ice" and cold water, and use only a light-pressure bandage. If it does not return spontaneously to its track, a lay-person must never attempt to re-align it. Carefully cool the knee-joint with "hot-ice." Do not apply a bandage of any kind, even an Ace bandage!

Follow-up Care

A doctor decides on an appropriate treatment plan. Systematic strengthening of the upper thigh muscles, under the guidance of a physical therapist, is most important, especially after a long pause in training or surgery (which may be performed after chronic dislocations). When the athlete is able to resume sports activities, the strength of the upper thigh and the circumference of the injured leg should be approximately identical to the uninjured, healthy upper thigh. If the thighs seem unequal in size have the doctor check the circumference of the muscle.

Knee supports can improve the function of the knee and provide the patient with a feeling of increased stability. However, they should not become dependent on them. Well-conditioned upper thigh muscles are vital for proper functioning.

Tip: If the problem continues, change to another sport.

NOTES

For more information about Marco Sport,
call Pro Nutrition at:
1-888-303-7668

NOTES

For more information about Wobenzym call:
1-888-4-VITAMINS
(1-888-484-8264)

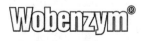

GENERAL

The human body is composed of 43.5% muscle. An athlete's body contains a considerably higher percentage. However, every human being has the same number of muscles. Training does not lead to increased muscle fibers and bundles (except within the heart) — they simply enlarge. The motor capacity of the billions of muscle fibers within our bodies is astounding; but only if that motor is in excellent starting and working condition. However, if the muscles are not warmed-up prior to exercise, they are prone to injury or damage. The most frequent muscle problems and treatment are described in the following sections.

MYOGELOSIS ("charley-horse")

"A muscle has seized up!" When this occurs, many athletes immediately quit a competition, instinctively doing the right thing. When, for example, the back of the upper thigh muscle feels tight (the most frequent localization), the muscle quickly loses its elasticity. The muscle bands shorten. If activity is continued, the muscle fiber may rupture from stretching beyond its limits.

Symptoms

A "charley-horse" causes an initial feeling of increased tension; it is generally not immediately painful, but additional stress causes additional pain. The athlete senses that the muscle has become less functional. Intuition should lead the athlete to discontinue training and seek immediate treatment. As a rule, no one except the injured person can properly evaluate the symptoms of a "charley-horse".

Occasionally, they can occur during sleep. One falls asleep comfortably and awakens with a hard leg muscle. This phenomenon is usually the result of an unfamiliar sleeping position, from lying cramped in a car or airplane, or when sleeping on an unfamiliar bed.

Causes

When one lies in bed the "wrong" way, an irritation of the nerve fibers extending from the spine is possible. If they happen to be motor fibers, which provide support for the upper thigh muscles, then the muscle tension may increase. Usually, pressure on the nerve fibers is the cause.

This can also happen from over-use of the lower back or the hips. New or improperly padded athletic shoes can bring about a "charley-horse."

First Aid

It is advisable to reduce the intensity of training. Discontinue all sports activities whenever the muscles seem tense. Gently stretch the affected area for 60 seconds. Perform warm-up exercises for the back (see "Practical Tips"). When stretching, take care not to push past the pain barrier. If muscles loosen up and the athlete wishes to resume activity, a slow, deliberate warm-up must be initiated. Stretch the weakened muscles for 7 seconds, follow-up with exercises which warm up all muscle groups, repeat 3 times per muscle group.

Follow-Up Care

1. Take frequent warm baths.
2. Do stretching after the bath, and loosen-up through general exercises.
3. Schedule a weekly massage from a massage therapist or physical therapist.
4. Place a "damp chamber" on the affected muscle. Dampen a cloth compress and place it flat on the injured area. Cover the entire area with plastic wrap and wrap it with a hand towel. Mild heat stimulates blood flow to the

capillaries. In most cases, the muscle tightness is relieved overnight.

Medications: Magnesium and Vitamin E supplements are helpful. (Consult your doctor for advice and dosage.)

MUSCLE BRUISES

Symptoms

All soccer players know about painful muscle bruises of the upper thigh. The bruise is usually caused by a kick, but skiers may get similar injuries from objects such as skis or ski-poles. The pain is acute, initially. The contusion (bruise) causes painful limitation of movements. A bruise develops in the muscle tissue. Small blood vessels are injured. A blood clot forms within the muscle, even when no outer signs of injury, such as an abrasion or discoloration, are noticeable on the skin.

A bruise does not necessarily indicate that the athlete should prematurely end a practice or competition. The injured player must determine that on the basis of the amount of pain being experienced. Use common sense. If the pain is severe, discontinue activity. Everything else depends on how fast the bruise heals. Small amounts of bleeding in the muscle produce small effects. Bruised tissue indicates increased bleeding. Activity should stop and a pressure bandage should be applied. If the pain remains or increases after a few hours, see your doctor.

Note: Injuries of the veins or arteries are also possible. Symptoms of injured major vessels include: constant pain even with the use of a pressure bandage, pale skin and a weak pulse. This requires immediate medical treatment (possibly surgery) at a hospital (see "Compartment Syndrome").

First Aid

First, apply "hot-ice" (ice water) with a cooling pressure bandage for 20 minutes. Submerge a sponge in ice-water; saturate an elastic bandage (1/2-inch wide) with ice water; wrap them together as a flat bandage around the injured area. On the upper thigh begin wrapping the bandage a little above the knee and finish it at the groin.

Do not use the bandage material too sparingly in this case! A too-short pressure bandage may act as a tourniquet for venous blood vessels and may lead to swelling of the limbs.

If the pressure bandage is not applied properly, oozing blood is guided into other areas. The blood vessels contract from the cold so that little blood is supplied to the area. To avoid this, use medium pressure and a sufficient number of Ace bandages to do the job.

Remember, the most important first measure: Quick cooling and compression. Position the injured leg above the level of the heart for at least 24 hours for a large bruise. (Position the injured leg at a 45° angle above the body while the patient is lying on his/her back.) The knee should be properly wrapped. Elevating the leg helps blood to return to the heart rather than pooling in the limb.

Follow-Up Care

Loosen the pressure bandage after 20-30 minutes. Observe the skin of the injured area; it will appear white after removal of the bandage. When the injured area appears red from the return of blood-flow (in about 2-4 minutes), apply a second pressure bandage. Repeat this process 3 or 4 times on the day of the accident. After that, apply ointment-bandages every 8 hours using Marco Sport Blue Gel or X-Cell-R-Aid ointment. For open skin injuries (wounds, abrasions, etc.), apply Betadine or Neosporin ointment on the first application (these preparations tend to cause less skin irritation).

Caution: Do not apply ice spray, heat or alcohol directly to the skin. These expand the blood vessels and would increase bleeding in the injured tissues. No massage in the first 24 hours. Do not use blood-thinning preparations (such as aspirin), which disturbs the natural clotting ability of blood and promotes secondary bleeding.

Conversely, lymphatic draining and electrical stimulation treatments done by a licensed physical therapist are ideal.

Compare the damaged leg with the healthy leg. If the injured area feels like "movable liquid", visit a doctor immediately for additional treatment.

Medications: To stimulate healing, anti-inflammatory preparations should be taken, such as Traumeel tablets, Bromalin capsules or Wobenzym. (Consult your doctor for advice and dosage.)

Treatment recommendation (from the 2nd day on): To decrease swelling rapidly, wrap the injured area with ointment-bandages (using Marco Sport Blue ointment). Alternate these with arnica tincture compresses (dilute: 2 Tbs. arnica tincture with ice-water). For persistent cases try aqua jogging or water therapy in a swimming pool or whirlpool for about 20 minutes.

For bruises on the leg, wrap bandages firmly around the injured area and move the leg in water for about 20 minutes. (The athlete may sit on the edge of the pool or be immersed while wearing a life-jacket.)

Perform isometrics, alternating tension-and-relaxation exercises. Elevate the slightly bent leg; tense for 7 seconds and relax for 10 seconds, for a total of about 20 minutes. After a 2-minute pause, repeat another series of 10 "reps".

Resumption of training: Normally, running practice may be resumed as early as the second day; however, the injured leg should be bandaged.

Prevention

Football, soccer and hockey players should wear shin-guards. Rub the upper thigh with massage oil or Vaseline before playing to allow attacks from the opposition to "slip off."

Hint: Teams should keep several Ace bandages and a bucket of ice-cold water at the coach's bench during games.

TRAUMATIC COMPARTMENT SYNDROME

Traumatic compartment syndrome is rare, but one of the most dangerous sports injuries. Caused by violent contact to a muscle compartment, a blow, kick, or thrust may cause considerable bleeding within the limbs. The area of the lower thigh is most likely to be affected.

At first, this may appear to be just a serious bruise, but if there is increasingly intense pain, along with profound swelling despite the use of appropriate first aid (see "First Aid" in the chapter "Muscle Bruises"), emergency treatment is required.

Every muscle is surrounded by a firm, supportive wrapping of tight connective tissue. If the bleeding does not stop, the pressure within the connective tissue rises precipitously because the fibrous tissue cannot expand.

The patient may experience intense to raging pain. Finally, the muscle receives no blood supply as pressure rises to near intolerable levels. Within a few hours there can be pressure damage to the muscle and nerve fibers in the affected area.

Muscle tissue begins to die and may leave the patient permanently disabled. See a doctor immediately! If possible, hyperbaric oxygen treatments should be performed at a hospital. A surgical procedure may be needed to release the constricting tissue and relieve the pressure.

Symptoms

Intense, increasingly severe pain in the injured area is a danger sign. Sometimes, peripheral sensory changes occur, such as a prickling sensation along the affected part or even loss of sensation.

First Aid

The trapped pressure must be relieved: Place the leg above the level of the heart and apply a pressure bandage with "hot-ice" for 20 minutes.

If pain increases with a pressure bandage, the bandage must be loosened or removed. In that case, apply a second pressure bandage with less tension and visit a doctor right away.

Follow-Up Care

To reduce swelling: Lymph-drainage may be necessary through "electro-stim" therapy (to be administered only by a licensed practitioner). To decrease trauma to the injured muscle elevate the leg at a 45° angle. Wrap with "hot-ice" and arnica tincture (2 Tbs. to 1 1/2 quarts of ice water); ointment- bandages, with Arnica gel or lotion, Neosporin, or Marco Sport Blue can be applied.

Medications: Bromalin capsules or Traumeel tablets are recommended. (Consult your doctor for advice and correct dosage.)

FUNCTIONAL COMPARTMENT SYNDROME

After muscle-straining activities (e.g. unaccustomed activity, hard floors, endurance-running, poor training conditions) a "charley-horse" may develop through the excessive lactic acid accumulation in the muscles. In this case, the athlete experiences rapidly increasing pain, along with symptoms of continuous muscle spasm. Additionally, there is a danger of a functional compartment syndrome. It is extremely rare but, like traumatic compartment syndrome, can be dangerous. Immediate treatment by a doctor is imperative. If there is doubt, a physician may choose to do an intra-muscular pressure measurement on the affected muscle. Ultrasound and CAT Scans are suitable diagnostic processes.

Symptoms

Minor motion may cause a cramp-like stabbing pain, and the sensation of a very severe muscle strain. The patient may experience diminished pain at rest and increased pain with motion.

Causes

Total physical exhaustion after ignoring the warning signs of the body, such as fatigue, "charley-horse" or muscular cramps, may cause this injury. It occurs predominantly in the lower thigh muscles. Due to continuous exertion, the muscles become excessively acidic, tension increases exponentially, and the muscle shortens and grows in circumference.

Consequences: Due to increasing interior pressure, the muscle's blood supply is reduced. Capillaries are neither supplied with blood nor drained. The muscle breaks down and pain occurs due to a lack of circulation. The muscle is still useable; but, with increasing pain exercise is not possible. Often, one can still walk, but can no longer run.

First Aid

Position the affected leg above the level of the heart. Apply "hot-ice" compresses. Hasten healing through positioning and cautious stretching. Grasp the leg with both hands and gently rub in the direction of the heart for about 7 minutes. Discuss electrotherapy treatments with your physician.

Medications: Wobenzym, Traumeel tablets and magnesium supplements. (Consult your doctor for advice and correct dosage.)

MUSCLE STRAIN/ OVER-STRETCHING

Nearly every athlete knows the feeling: a quick step or fast motion — and suddenly one feels a cramp-like pain in the upper thigh or the calf. In recent years, the number of cases involving muscle strain have noticeably diminished due to improved warm-up exercises and stretching before training or competition (see "Practical Tips"). However, muscle-strain is still among the most common of sport-related complaints. Although there is no acute pain, any additional exertion of the inflamed muscle may cause a muscle-fiber rupture or even a torn muscle.

Over-stretching and the tearing of a muscle are, according to many years of observation and experience, two basically different injuries. Over-stretching deals with a disturbance of muscular function, a "derailment" of the regulation of muscular tension. Unlike a muscle fiber rupture, no fibers are torn, nor is there any bleeding or any localized center of pain.

Ignoring the complaints of a muscular strain/over-stretch often leads, however, to a fiber-rupture or even a muscle tear. With appropriate therapy, the athlete can have the full use of the injured area after 3-4 days.

Symptoms

A stressed or over-stretched muscle is usually not acutely noticeable, in contrast to a torn muscle. At first, an increasing generalized discomfort is felt in a muscle. This is followed by a pulling sensation, tension, and finally, cramp-like pains.

The athlete usually does not want to quit. However, increasing pain in the muscle may cause a feeling of anxiety, and the athlete fears that continuing will lead to "tearing something." Every athlete with an over-stressed muscle reacts the same. The person tries to loosen-up by shaking the affected leg. No relief. The longer the over-stretched muscle continues to be used, the worse the athlete feels.

Causes

Inadequate preparation before training or sports is usually the cause of the strain. After a generous warm-up of the muscles, another brief warming-up stretch should follow to allow all the significant muscles (for the activity) to be stretched.

In warm weather, the danger of over-stretching is greater because you perspire more and lose fluids and minerals — both of which are important for the optimal functioning of the muscles.

Additional causes are: poor overall conditioning of the body, on-going problems such as genetic conditions of the feet, inflamed areas of the body, such as tonsillitis, infected sinuses, or abscessed teeth, flu or gout.

Field conditions also can cause such muscle problems. If

you've prepared yourself for a hard surface and have to play on grass later on, the muscles cannot adjust themselves quickly to the new ground. Therefore, the danger of over-stretching increases during the readjustment phase. Try to anticipate field conditions and prepare appropriately.

Note: The muscles of a professional athlete react to a change of ground with much more sensitivity than the muscles of an amateur player.

The wrong type of shoe may also cause over-stretching. Quality sports shoes cost more, but they preserve the joints, tendons and muscles with stabilizing soles and innersoles. This also can be said for the correct choice of cleats. For instance, we recommend knob-shoes for training. Cleats should only be used in competition and on grassy fields.

First Aid

The most important factor in the treatment of an over-stretched muscle is the "relaxation" of the muscle. The injured area is first wrapped for 20 minutes with a "hot-ice" pressure bandage. Then, re-evaluate the injury. A sponge can be saturated with ice water and wrapped around the injured muscle with an ice-water-permeated Ace bandage (3 inches wide). Dampen the bandage with more ice water or place a cold pack on it as needed. Do not treat the area with heat or warming ointments. In most cases, the pain is dispelled during the first 20 minutes, because the cold has a relaxing effect.

If discomfort persists, or increases, you must consider the diagnosis of a muscle fiber tear. The symptoms of over-stretching and fiber tear are described in quite similar terms by athletes without prior injuries.

After the "hot-ice" pressure bandage, stretch the muscle within the pain-free zone. Begin cautiously with mild, gentle stretching. Stretch the affected muscle for 7-10 seconds, then allow for rest, and stretch again. Repeat these exercises 10-15 times. Following this, apply an ointment-bandage such as Marco Sport Blue overnight.

Medications: Vitamin E and Magnesium supplements are helpful. (See your doctor for advice and dosage.) Pain-killing remedies and ointments are not recommended. A clear head enables the athlete to monitor the healing process and report changes to the doctor or therapist.

Follow-Up Care

First day after the injury: Stretching exercises may be attempted as described under First Aid. Try a slow jog (within endurance), or training on a stationary bicycle. Continue for up to 20 minutes, but avoid exercising to the point of pain.

Important: Do not attempt motions requiring take-off power! The muscle must be gradually re-trained to assume function, afterward, "hot-ice" compresses for reduction of renewed muscle tension. Also recommended are ultrasound applications, electro-therapy, and massage. (Consult a doctor or licensed physical therapist.)

Second day: Do stretching exercises (as on the previous day). Train for 20 minutes each morning and afternoon, jogging within endurance — no sprints! After running, apply "hot-ice" compresses. After the second training session, recuperate by stretching and exercises (as directed by the physical therapist).

Third day: Stretch in the morning and afternoon, followed by 20 minutes of jogging at a slightly increased speed.

Additionally, proceed as on the second day.

Fourth day: Generally, normal training can be resumed.

Important: Make absolutely sure that all exercises do not cause pain.

Prevention

Over-stretching can be avoided by an appropriate warm-up (see "Practical Tips"). For various "ball" sports, a 20-minute warm-up is recommended. For tennis, 15 minutes are appropriate. Even a golfer should warm up for at least 10 minutes before the first stroke. The body and muscles must be slowly turned-up to "working temperature" before a full range of activities are undertaken.

We notice again and again that many cases of muscle over-stretching are connected to improper clothing during the warming-up. Many people warm-up in their training gear, and then put plastic jackets and pants over them to continue the warm-up in the shortest time. Shortly before the competition, they take off these outfits. This is a mistake! The skin and muscles suffer from a sudden drop in temperature. As soon as one begins to perspire slightly during warm-up, they are advised to take off heavy outerwear, and the additional warm-up should be completed under competitive conditions. However, this does not apply to sports which require take-off power or sprinting (brief, high-exertion efforts).

Hint: Wearing a net-shirt under the tricot (team "jersey"), will prevent absorption of perspiration by the uniform. Proper nutrition, lots of liquids, and minerals (see "Practical Tips") are important to avoid over-stretching.

RUPTURED MUSCLE-FIBER

The rapid healing of muscle-fiber-ruptures has caused heated discussion recently. The rapid recovery of National Soccer player, Juergen Klinsmann, who returned to the European Master Competition 1996 in England after just 7 days, amazed many. As a rule, the treatment for a muscle-fiber-rupture takes at least 10 days from the date of injury to the return of the athlete.

In the case of Klinsmann, a series of "fortunate circumstances" made his rapid recuperation possible. It was a unique case which cannot be considered "normal." The same level of around-the-clock medical care and physical therapy is impossible for the majority of athletes.

Symptoms

How to recognize a muscle-fiber-rupture? In contrast to the over-stretched muscle, in which a cramp-like pain develops, the injured area in a muscle-fiber-rupture causes sudden, acute pain which prevents movement.

Depending on the severity and extent of the injury, it is experienced as a piercing or dull stab — the larger the rupture, the blunter the pain.

No hematoma (bruise) is usually visible. If any bleeding is noticeable, a muscle rupture is suspected.

Causes

Muscle-fiber-ruptures usually come about during or after extreme exertion, such as repeated long sprints, whenever the muscle is over-stressed and/or loaded with lactic acid (a by-product of muscle metabolism). This injury, like over-stretching, can also be caused by an insufficient warming-up, poor training and conditioning, or a rapid loss of minerals due to heavy perspiring. Insufficiently-healed prior injuries and/or disturbances in coordination may also be involved. In an extended sense, metabolic disturbances (gout or inflamed tonsils or teeth) may also exacerbate this tendency.

First Aid

Immediate, correct first aid of a muscle-fiber-rupture is decidedly important. Bleeding must be immediately limited by pressure and cold. Within 10 minutes after the injury, at the latest, apply a cold pressure bandage with "hot-ice." Afterward, the body begins its self-regulation at the site of the injury. This has an undesirable effect on the healing process, since each minute lost before treatment requires an additional day of "down" time.

How to apply the Pressure Bandage: Relax the injured muscle and place in an inclined position (e.g. for a fiber rupture in the upper or lower thigh, the mildly bent knee should be placed above the level of the hip). Place a sponge saturated with ice water on the injury and then wrap with a "hot-ice" bandage (such as a 3-inch-wide Ace bandage, saturated with ice water) which is wrapped with heavy tension. Allow it to remain for only 20 minutes and keep saturating it with ice water.

After 20 minutes, loosen the pressure bandage. Otherwise, the muscle metabolism becomes disturbed. This could cause considerable additional damage. By removing the pressure bandage, the muscle is again provided with blood, oxygen and nutrients.

After a pause of 4-5 minutes, apply another pressure bandage with "hot-ice" for another 20 minutes. Repeat this process 3-4 times, maintaining the pauses. During this time, do not exercise the muscle.

In the case of serious injuries, such as ruptured-muscular-fascia (muscle covering) or a ruptured muscle, the bleeding should subside after only 3 hours as a general rule.

Important: The patient should subsequently take a shower with the pressure bandage on. Without the pressure bandage, the warm water may bring too much heat from the outside and provoke secondary bleeding. As follow-up care we advise a cooling ointment bandage, such as Marco Sport Blue or Neosporin ointment, for the next 8 hours.

Note: With all injuries, it is fundamental for the injured person to abstain from alcohol of any kind for the first 24 hours. Alcohol disturbs fluid regulation and causes the injury to absorb water, and swelling of the tissue (edema) will be worse.

Medications: Traumeel tabs. or drops, Wobenzym (10 tabs. 2x daily), zinc (l tab. 2x daily), Vitamin C (1g daily), Vitamin E (800mg daily). (Consult your doctor.)

Important: Consult your doctor before taking any pain-relief tablets. Overuse of medication may allow further injury to the area if the senses are dulled. This prevents protection of the injury, and also delays the healing process.

Follow-up Care

Additional treatment and rehabilitation must be undertaken by a doctor and a physical therapist. The following therapeutic procedure has proven effective:

1. Assist in the rapid healing of the wound (ruptured fibers) as quickly as possible, with freedom of pain (without analgesic substances) by following a daily regimen of cooling ointment-bandages and elevating the injured part. All symptoms of injury, such as shortening of the injured

muscle in which the ruptured fiber is located, are treated and repaired. With diligent treatment, the muscle fibers can be brought into better condition than before the injury. This occurs with conscientious professional care, such as drainage of the bruise and prevention of circulatory problems. Shiatsu and deep massages of non-injured muscle areas may be advised. One proceeds slowly, and the ruptured fiber is on a "recess" during the first five days. Also helpful are mobilization of the adjoining areas, passive and active stretching of muscles within the pain-free-zone, electro-therapy, and infiltration of medication into the injured muscle (performed by a licensed practitioner). We advise the use of ointment-bandages during the night.

2. Exercise and retraining of the remaining adjacent muscles which take over the function of the injured, not-yet-fully-healed muscles.
3. From the 5th day on: In addition to physical therapy measures, a jogging trial is recommended for the 5th day. Begin with a light, continuous jog for 20 minutes. On the next two days, if possible, jog two times for 20 minutes, moving with increasing intensity, but not causing pain.
4. From the 8th day on, accelerated runs are acceptable. From the 10th day forward, sprints and conditioning exercises can be accomplished, if no discomfort is felt.
5. Soccer and football players may resume their ball training when all running exercises can be performed without any pain; otherwise, there is danger of a relapse.

Practical Rule: If pain is felt in the injured area during the first exercises, you must stop training. Otherwise, the healing process will be delayed. With premature stress and a renewed injury, a longer rehabilitation phase is likely.

Important: After every therapeutic measure, the injured muscle must be cooled with "hot-ice" treatment in order to avoid possible overheating of the area. After each training session, cool-down measures, stretching, and active regeneration are mandatory (see "Practical Tips").

Prevention (See Over-stretching.)

MUSCLE CRAMPS

The muscle cramp is among those complaints that can be relieved quickly, either by the athlete or with the aid of a coach. After over-stressing a muscle group for some time, the athlete feels acute pain — most frequently in the calves, upper thighs or toes. The athlete is unable to continue running. Extreme discomfort, along with swelling lead to painful limitation of movement.

Symptoms

An athlete may report acute, intense pain in the muscles, severe limitation of movement, possible immobility, or extreme pressure in the affected muscle area.

Causes

The reason for a muscle cramp lies in a disturbance of the muscle metabolism. There are a series of conditions responsible for this: general tiredness, stress, poor physical conditioning, tight clothing, socks or shin guards that may cut off blood flow and cause calf muscle areas circulatory disturbances. Naturally, these occur more frequently during the summer than in the winter, since higher temperatures lead to the loss of mineral salts. Additionally, varicose veins, disturbances in the area of the lower back, wrong or poorly fitting shoes, or foot problems — all of these can lead to nasty muscle cramps.

First Aid

For calf cramps, it is important to immediately stretch the affected muscle. Set the foot on the ground without stretching the knee-joint of the affected leg; rather let it form an approximately 90° angle. Pull the toes toward you with both hands, if possible. Hold this position for 20 seconds. Repeat this process 3-4 times.

If this does not relieve the spasm, a companion or partner can help in the following way: The "patient" lies down on his/her stomach. The affected lower thigh is placed at a right angle to the upper thigh and the toes are pressed in the direction of the knee. If tolerable, hold this stretch for 20 seconds, and after a brief respite, repeat 3-4 times. If the spasm is relieved, the "patient" can produce counter-pressure with the toes pressed against the hand of the helper.

Subsequently, rub the calf and the hollow of the knee (fossa) of the affected leg with a sponge dipped in ice water. This is recommended to improve the circulation in the affected area.

For cramps of the back of the upper thigh muscle, gently and passively stretch the cramped and shortened muscle. Bend the upper body forward while standing on the unaffected leg. This position should be held until the spasm fades. Following this, rub the upper thigh with an ice-water-saturated sponge.

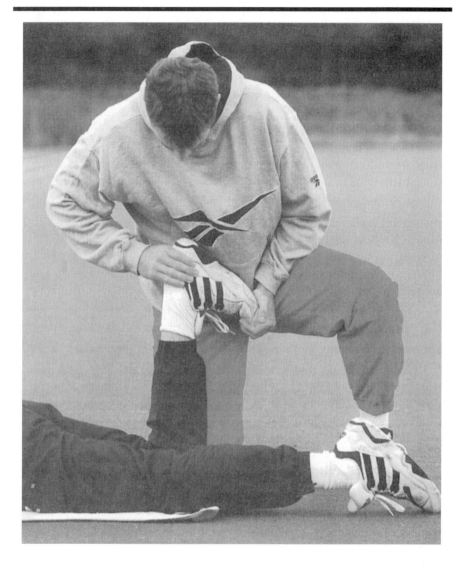

SPASM IN THE CALF:
The athlete lies on his abdomen. The leg is bent at the knee. A colleague presses the tip of the foot firmly toward the knee, holding this position for 15-20 seconds. Then release the pressure for about 10 seconds. Repeat the process 2-3 times.

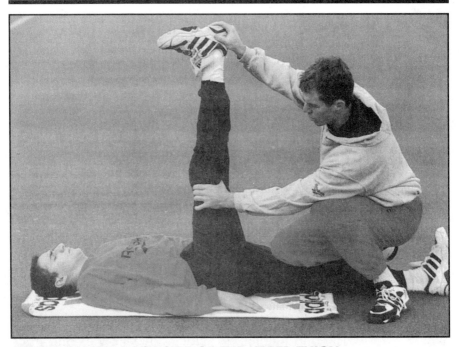

SPASM ON THE BACK SIDE OF THE UPPER THIGH:
The athlete lies on his back. A colleague kneels lightly on the stretched-out leg; the raised leg is held at the knee, pressed toward the torso, and held for 15-20 seconds. Repeat the process 2-3 times.

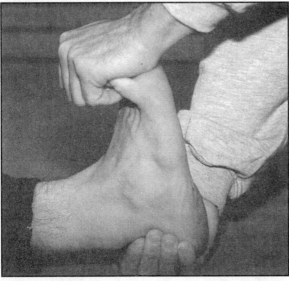

SOLVING A SPASM IN THE TOES:
The heel of the foot is held by one hand. With the other hand, press the toes back over the top of the foot. Hold for 15-20 seconds. Repeat 2-3 times.

Follow-Up Care

Use a whirlpool with warm water, take salt tablets, and use sports drinks.

Prevention

Always perform stretching and exercises before training or competition. Stay in good condition. Do not carry fitness exercises too far. Brief intervals are preferable for training. A series of exercises for strength (such as 10x 7-10 exercise repetitions) accomplished, with 2 minutes of rest between "reps" are preferable to 50 exercises in an unbroken sequence.

Replace fluids during competitive events and during breaks, chiefly through fresh water with little or no carbonation. Try small portions of lukewarm tea with lemon (for better absorption by the body). After the sports event, a mixture of apple juice and mineral water is very tasty and helpful in replacing electrolytes and trace elements lost through perspiration. Before taking mineral salt tablets or mineral drinks, confer with an expert, since quality from product to product varies greatly.

Important: Do not consume ice-cold drinks or alcohol!

If the athlete experiences low-back-spasm, an examination of the lower back by a specialist is advised, along with laboratory testing of blood samples.

Hint: Knee-high socks and shin guards should never be fastened with elastic or rubber bands, but only with rolled gauze or loose strips of tape.

SORE MUSCLES

Many athletes, unfortunately, still believe antiquated and false notions that muscle soreness after stressful training is proof of hard work. However, sore muscles are caused by damaged tissues in the area of the muscle fibers. They do not indicate a serious injury, but they are avoidable through well-planned and executed training. Hikers usually experience soreness after an exceptionally challenging descent.

Symptoms

Following a strenuous exercise, a pause in regular training, or after insufficient preparation, the muscles feel tired (e.g. heavy legs). Coordination is poor. Following exercise, muscle pain occurs. It may be incapacitating for some.

Causes

Through excessive demands, or unusual positioning, as well as using the legs as "shock-absorbers" e.g., as in descending a mountain, down-hill runs, etc., lactic acid and metabolic "debris" are deposited in the muscles. This disturbs the circulation and causes tissue irritation. Climbing a mountain usually does not lead to sore muscles, but rather to muscle tiredness.

With fatigue and a lack of coordination, the danger of injury rises. For example, in a long tennis match, which you absolutely want to finish, you can easily stumble over your own feet or "knick" a muscle. Without the stabilization of the joints by the muscles, the danger of a ruptured ligament is increased.

First Aid

To eliminate waste-matter quickly and decrease muscle soreness, active and passive exercises must be done promptly. It would be more difficult to obtain the same results on the following day.

Despite tiredness, every professional or amateur athlete should develop the habit of performing a cool-down routine after each event. First, gently stretch the stressed muscles (see "Practical Tips"). This is the way to prevent painful muscle soreness.

It is also recommended to enjoy an easy slow jog and, if possible, to exercise for 15-20 minutes on a stationary bicycle without exerting much effort. In order to avoid heat accumulation, be sure to wear "breathable" fabrics.

Also helpful is a relaxing tub bath in 98-102º F warm water for 10-15 minutes. Try adding bath salts or a handful of table salt.

Using the sauna is soothing, but only for 6-8 minutes at a reduced temperature (120-130º F). Before the sauna, be sure to take in ample fluids; never enter it dehydrated. Subsequently, rest is appropriate, possibly with a regenerating massage by an experienced therapist (but avoid massage if touch is painful).

What to do if sore muscles occur nevertheless? Rigid muscles should be carefully cooled-down. One can try a light jog. Motion frequently improves with warming of the muscles. The length of the training will be different from person-to-person. As a rule, you should run until you feel a renewed fatigue of the muscles. Never repeat the activity that caused the soreness originally.

If it is a serious case of muscle soreness, water therapy is recommended, including aqua jogging, bicycling, or massage by a therapist.

Follow-Up Care

To mitigate the pain, you could take Aspirin + C. Also one can add Bromalin or Wobenzym (2 tablets 3x daily).

Hint: During power-training: Do not practice forcefully. A 2-5 minute pause is recommended after each group of 10 "reps" of an exercise before beginning the next series.

Mountain Climbers: We especially recommend that those with low back pain or arthritis of the spine hike up the mountain and take the cable-car down! If you must descend the mountain on foot, use a cane or walking stick.

NOTES

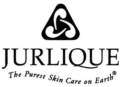

For more information about Jurlique Call:
1-800-854-1110

JURLIQUE
The Purest Skin Care on Earth®

GROIN INJURIES

The body's weakest area is the groin. Its unprotected location from the pelvic bones to the pubic bone makes it especially vulnerable to injuries during sports activities such as sprints, soccer or football. Demands on groin structures are often excessive, sometimes resulting in long, drawn-out injuries. Problems may include hernias and muscles ruptures, as well as secondary difficulties in other areas of the body. Injuries of the groin and thighs may be caused by other factors, such as problems with the hips or back, which can project pain into the groin.

Non-professionals should not attempt diagnosis of injuries. Only a doctor, together with an experienced sports physical therapist, can make an accurate diagnosis and create a treatment plan. Whenever a groin injury occurs, you should consult your physician immediately.

Symptoms

Upon injury, the affected athlete usually feels a pulling pain in the area of the groin and abdominal muscles; the athlete may also feel a "burning" or "stabbing" pain, along with the feeling of being unable to perform normal motions. Pain originating from these injuries may radiate into the muscles on the inside of the upper thigh which limits freedom of motion. The athlete may also experience "pulling" pain running from the lower back (S.I. joint) to the hip and into the groin, and sometimes beyond that into other muscles — depending on the seriousness and cause of injury. Intense pain in these areas is typical of groin injuries resulting from fast movements or lunging forward.

Signs of groin injury are obvious to the onlooker. The athlete is seen pressing the area with the hand or using a protective posture (an automatic bending forward). These are definite signs that the athlete is experiencing pain and are symptomatic of the beginning stage of a ruptured groin. As a consequence of weakness of the diagonal pelvic muscle and related tendon (from either congenital causes or resulting from injury), the tendon canal widens. Extreme tension along the abdominal muscles and high pressure inside the abdomen while sprinting or kicking may cause intense pain. Coughing and sneezing may also cause considerable pain. In the case of a ruptured groin, the muscle is injured due to increased pressure within the abdomen. In this case, sneezing or kicking can result in severe, "strangulating" pain if organs are entrapped within the muscle separation.

Causes

Insufficient recuperation after high-stress training and play during sports such as football, handball, tennis, volleyball, ice-speed-skating, or during short or medium distance races may produce an injury. Another cause is exceptionally high pressure or injuries to the pelvic muscles (adductors). For example, injuries may occur from infrequent training, incorrect abdominal exercises changing from soft to hard floors in the winter, or training on unfamiliar floors in the gym, or insufficient warm-ups and stretching. Poor posture while sitting for long periods in buses and airplanes may result in problems.

Inflammation from other locations in the body can cause or be a contributory factor to problems in the groin area (such as infection of dental roots, tonsils, sinuses, prostate, or testicles). A painful lymph node (gland) swelling of the upper thigh may occur from bacterial inflammation. The swelling may be a secondary effect of infected abrasions, blisters or athletes foot of the affected leg. These may require treatment with antibiotics. Again, consult your physician.

First Aid

If the athlete feels only a mild "pulling" sensation, the sports activity may be continued at a later date — after some initial treatment. First, perform careful stretching exercises within the pain-free-zone (see "Practical Tips"). If the pain increases, cool the area immediately with "hot ice" (wet a sponge or cloth with ice water) and place it on the injured area for 15-20 minutes. If the groin pain radiates from the back, a "capsicum patch" on the lower spine (check with your pharmacist) usually brings relief. In the case of very painful or chronic groin injuries, consult your doctor.

The athlete must carefully follow recommended treatment and not resume training too early. Be careful not to perform extensive abdominal-muscle exercises before groin pain has subsided for a few days. Doing so would further irritate the groin.

If other muscle injuries, such as a "pulled muscle" or a ruptured-muscle-fiber in the abdomen or thigh area is diagnosed, previously recommended treatment may be applied. (See chapter on "Ruptured Muscle Fiber").

For a "charley-horse", the care described in the corresponding chapter is useful.

Medications: Do not use pain killers as the doctor needs a precise, clear description of the pain.

Follow-up Care

When groin problems result from a "charley-horse", medicated baths improve circulation in the affected area and help lessen discomfort. There are several medicated bath products available in health food stores. Batherapy is one such product. Consult your doctor for suggestions.

Pour the recommended amount of the product into water

which is about 100º F and soak for 15-20 minutes. Afterwards, wrap-up in a clean bath sheet and a wool blanket. Rest for 20 minutes.

After resting, gently perform stationary stretching exercises within the pain-free-zone (see photos following). At night, place bandages on the abdominal muscles to relax the musculature. For example, using Marco Sport Green Ointment, dampen a gauze or Kerlex compress, spread ointment generously on the bandage and place on the injured area. Finally, wrap with an Ace bandage. Secure it with strips of bandage tape.

When the groin problems originate from the back, one needs to apply a "damp chamber" or a "fire packing" with capsicum ointment to the painful area of the back.

When there are painful or unrelenting complaints, treatment must be administered by an experienced physical therapist. Suggested are: Manual therapy through massage of back, buttocks and upper thigh; therapeutic baths with bath salts, ultrasound, or underwater massage.

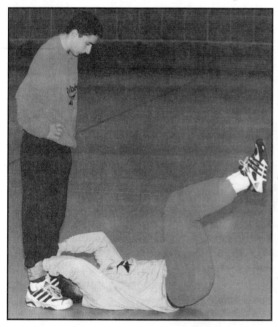

THE CLASSIC ABDOMINAL EXERCISE, OMITTING THE HIP-JOINT MUSCLE:
The athlete lies on his back, hands grasping the ankles of the partner. Hip and knees are bent at a 90º angle. The pelvis is raised through the tensing of the abdominal muscle. Duration depends on the condition of training.

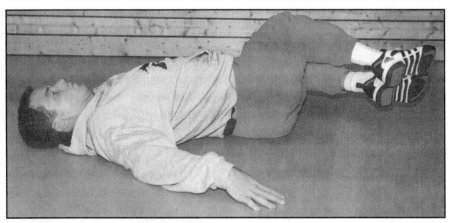

***EXERCISE FOR THE DIAGONAL
ABDOMINAL MUSCULATURE:***
*The athlete lies on his back with arms spread out from the body
for stabilization. The legs are close together at an angle and fall
to the left and right sides, keeping slightly above the floor.
Duration depends on the condition of training.*

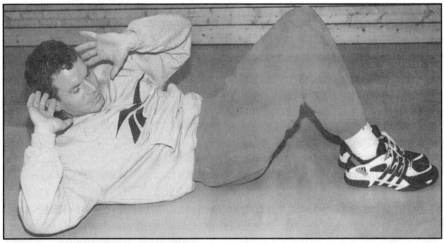

***EXERCISE FOR THE DIAGONAL
ABDOMINAL MUSCULATURE:***
*The legs are bent and remain in this position while the upper
body moves alternately toward the opposite knee. Duration
depends on the condition of training.*

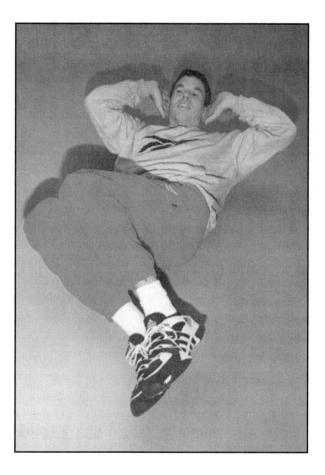

***EXERCISE FOR THE ENTIRE
ABDOMINAL MUSCULATURE:***
*With knees bent, hip angled, and straight
upper body, place the fingertips on the
ears. The knees fall to one side and the
upper body moves straight upward.*

Prevention

This consists of regular and consistent warm-ups of all involved muscle groups and correct training of the abdominal muscles (see photos and instructions on pages 72-74). Avoid training on slippery surfaces! Choose the proper shoes. Practice as little as possible (or not at all) with spikes or cleats. For training indoors, select shoes with shock-absorbing soles. After training and sports, take refreshing baths in luke-warm water of about 100º F.

Pay attention to body hygiene; foot fungus can, under certain circumstances, lead to swelling of the lymph nodes (glands) of the groin. This may be avoided by wearing shower sandals in the locker room. After a shower, carefully towel-dry the feet, or use a hairdryer, paying special attention to the spaces between the toes. Wear fresh socks daily!

Although it often seems bothersome (and one must overcome that), the rule for all athletes before training and games should be: 20 minutes of warming-up and stretching exercises. These are a necessary investment that will make you better prepared physically. It is noteworthy that gymnasts are generally spared from sustaining groin injuries — this is the result of thoroughly exercising the entire body.

NOTES

Hastings House Book Publishers
Tel: 203-838-4083
Fax: 203-838-4084

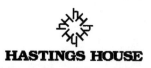

HASTINGS HOUSE

PAIN IN THE LOWER BACK / SCIATICA

It is incredible what the spinal column must tolerate, especially during sports. The spine is the body's axis and is challenged by certain situations. It can support up to a ton of pressure for short periods. Functional disturbances in the area of the lumbar spine, as well as signs of wear, are the frequent consequence. They make themselves known in the form of pain in the lower back (which may be excruciating). Pain can also radiate to other areas.

Back pain is the expression of the extensive lack of exercise in modern civilization.

Symptoms

Back pain announces itself through painful, acute limitation of motion in all directions, such as in bending forward, bending sideways, or turning. Symptoms usually include a "pulling", "stabbing" or "cramp-like" pain, which may radiate to the groin (lower abdomen), the buttocks, or the leg. The origin of the pain can also shift around and at times is difficult to pinpoint.

Typically, the injured athlete can only move with great effort and takes on a stiffly defensive posture to avoid additional pain. In acute cases, even getting up is impossible without someone's assistance. In the vernacular, this is known as "lumbago."

An acute pain which radiates into the back of the leg is called "sciatica."

Note: If there is a feeling of numbness, muscular weakness, or apparent paralysis, promptly visit a doctor.

Symptoms of Sciatica

During strenuous or sudden motion, the athlete feels an acute "stabbing" pain in the lower back (from lifting something with a bent back during a turning motion), which nearly renders him immobile. The athlete feels as though he/she has been struck by lightening and remains bent over, unable to straighten up.

However, discomfort may not be felt for hours after intense stress, when a minor movement causes "Sciatica" (pain radiating to the leg).

Dislocation of the Disk

If the pain radiates from the lower spine via the leg and down to the foot in such a way that the athlete can trace the path of the pain with a finger, it is most likely referred pain. This may be caused by a problem disk (involving, for example, pain referred to the lower groin, buttocks, or outer side of upper and lower thigh). Coughing and pressure increases the pain.

The following test is an indicator for the lay-person: If the affected athlete bends the upper body to the pain-free side and the pain increases, a disk may be indicated.

Causes of Pain in the Lower Back

Causes may include misuse or over-stressing of a section of the spine, a damaged disk, malformation of the spine, or pressure from poorly conditioned muscles of the pelvis and spinal column. Weakness of the back, muscle spasm or muscle injuries, or having one leg shorter than the other can also contribute to problems.

Additional causes: These may include violent trauma (being hit, kicked, or falling), unique movements, such as those used in spear tossing, discus hurling, golf, trampoline use or diving. Poor technique, such as in serving the ball while hunched forward in a tennis match, lifting weights from the lower spine, for example. Also, drafts and cooling-off while perspiring can be contributory causes of considerable pain in the sacral area.

First Aid

A few days of rest and good care are usually enough to eliminate pain. This is preferably done while sitting in a chair and keeping the hips and knees at approximately right angles.

Pain in the lumbar area requires warmth. A bath at about 98-102º F, with the addition of circulation-enhancing bath salts is helpful.

Use "fire-packing." Place a hot pack or heating pad on a sheet. Cover this with plastic and a towel saturated with hot water. The patient lies on the back and pulls the sheet together over the abdomen with the packing lying close to the body. Allow the warmth to take effect for 20-30 minutes. The legs should be lightly-wrapped and bent at the knees. To increase the heat effect even more, one can rub heat-producing ointments into the area such as Marco Sport Red.

Alternatively: Use irradiation of the painful area with an infrared lamp from a medical supply store or pharmacy. Sit down on a stool, with a damp cloth covering the back. Place a large, dry towel over it (one that is large enough to be fastened around the abdomen). Place the infrared lamp about 12-16 inches from the back and allow the heat to penetrate for about 20 minutes.

After the heat therapy, stretch and loosen the back, as shown in the picture on page 81.

Overnight, it is also recommended to place a capsicium patch on the painful area.

Alternatively, the affected area can be rubbed with Bengay ointment. Another very effective treatment is to warm up a container of Flexall or Cramergesic salve in hot water, shake it well, and generously apply it to absorbent gauze. Place the pack on the painful area. Wrap it with a large towel, and have the patient lie on his/her back.

Important: Have the patient assume a comfortable position. Place supports under the lower thighs so that the hip and knee-joints are bent at approximately right angles (an inclined arrangement). Allow the packing to remain until no more heat is felt. Following that, the patient should take a shower and dress warmly.

Hint: After heat therapy, dry the skin thoroughly, allowing time for all perspiration to evaporate, and advise avoiding drafts. Suggest cotton clothing or a special abdominal binder (such as one made of angora wool) in order to retain the heat.

In damp and cold, windy weather, protection should be provided by using Neoprene kidney protectors (as for jogging). We recommend wearing a cotton undershirt for absorption of perspiration and skin protection.

Medications: Aspirin + C, magnesium supplement, Vitamin E as well as Vitamin B. (Consult with your doctor.)

Note: If there is no perceptible improvement after a few days of following the recommended measures, a doctor should be seen. Any sense of numbness or signs of paralysis require medical attention. When there is acute lower back pain, only professionals should touch the painful area.

ROCKING EXERCISE FOR LOOSENING THE INDIVIDUAL VERTEBRAL SEGMENTS AND FOR STRETCHING THE BACK MUSCULATURE: **The knees are pulled close to the chest and clasped by the hands. The upper body is pressed close to the upper thigh with the head near the knees. The athlete rocks on the rounded back about 10-15 times, without motion in the hip joint.**

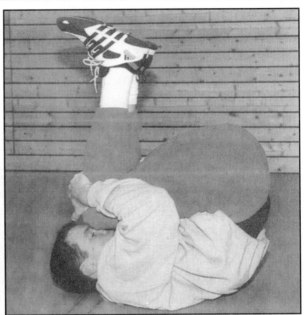

Follow-Up Care

After the applications of heat, simple exercises may be started for stretching and loosening of the muscles. In addition to the illustrated exercises, the following measures are also quite effective: Lie on the back with knees bent, pull up the knees as far as possible and lean to the left and right as you turn the head to the opposite side each time. (Repeat 10-15 times with equal rest periods.) Advise stretching in a sitting position on a stool: Clasp your hands at the nape of the neck and press the left elbow to the right knee and then the right elbow to the left knee. Also helpful is stretching of the lower back through "hanging out" (leaning over a railing or banister) with a slight dangling of legs. If increased pain occurs, however, it should be discontinued.

MOBILIZATION OF THE SPINAL COLUMN IN THE AREA OF THE LUMBAR SPINE AND THE LOWER THORACIC VERTEBRAL COLUMN:
The athlete sits on a chair with a back support and arm rests, with legs slightly separated and feet firmly on the floor. Now twist the upper body with the help of the arm muscles against the pelvis while the hands firmly hold the chair arm. Apply this exercise in both directions and repeat 5-10 times.

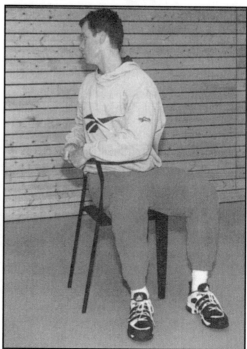

Note: Be cautious with traction devices in the home: these should be used only after demonstration by a physical therapist.

Important: Exercises may be done only within the pain-free-zone and only to the point of fatigue. This point of tiredness is reached when the muscles begin to "tremble." This should conclude the exercises.

When totally free from pain, you may change to exercises for stabilization of the back and abdominal muscles:

Exercise 1: Lying on the back, pull the toes upward and raise the legs from the hip evenly upward. Hold both arms above the head. To use more energy, press the hands against a wall (about 7-10 seconds holding, followed by 7-10 seconds of release). Repeat 8-10 times.

Exercise 2: Lying on back with knees bent and heels pressed into the floor, pull the toes up. Place arms next to the head on the floor, and press down. Then the arms are placed so that the back of the hands touch the floor. Now, raise the head and hold for 7-10 seconds, brief pause 7-10 seconds, then repeat 8-10 times.

Exercise 3: Mobilization of the lower back: Take a "four-legged position" and walk, then raise the back like a cat and return to the starting position. Repeat the exercise about 8-10 times.

If you have time and a swimming pool: Take a daily swim (using a backstroke), whenever possible, at a comfortable water temperature (at least 82° F). Being cold (which leads to an unwanted shortening of the muscles) indicates that swimming should be discontinued. We advise against the breast stroke because the head bends the neck. The lower back may easily slip into an arched position during the leg stroke. This leads to stress of the inter-vertebral disks and the vertebral (back) joints.

Hint: After swimming, it is important to dress immediately and dry the hair. With wet dripping hair, the nape of the neck remains damp and cold for an extended time. This cold may cause an acutely stiff neck.

Prevention

Here, too, prevention is better and simpler than healing.

Training: Improve the flexibility of the back through daily exercises. A well-exercised muscle is the best protection for a hard-working lower spine. However, be cautious with power training. Make sure a "clean" technique is used. Lifting weights with a bent lower spine is not advisable. We advise doing as the weight lifter does: Go into the squat position and with a straight and firm back, lift while using the legs.

Posture: Positioning is usually the cause of the development of a "slipped disk". Work on improving posture, especially while seated. A reclining position is ideal: Slant the seat of the chair by using a foam rubber wedge. This forces the muscles of the back against the back of the chair and maintains a good position while sitting. An alternative positioning aid is the "Pezi-Ball" (from a health supply store).

Weight: Avoid becoming overweight! "Heavyweights" should realize how much of an extra burden they carry.

Clothing: In rainy weather, clothes for training should be wind and water repellent and at the same time be able to absorb perspiration. A net-shirt next to the skin is ideal with a cotton shirt or a tricot (jersey) over it. The outer layer should be a training jacket. Materials which do not allow any air circulation are unsuitable and can lead to over-heating.

Shoes: If feelings of fatigue and pain in the feet or spine develop, have the feet checked out. Pay attention to sensible shoes and inlays.

Bed: A spinal column that is stressed during the day should be able to relax on a "medium firmness" sleeping surface. The mattress must not be sloping or sagging (support with a firm innerspring or wooden platform). A good mattress should support the curves of the body such as the buttocks, hips, and shoulders.

NECK PAIN / NECK STIFFNESS

Neck pain generally develops due to a disturbed function of the individual sections of the cervical and upper thoracic spine. It may radiate into the shoulders, arms, back, and the back of the head.

Symptoms

Turning the head is associated with intense pain due to the movement (kinesalgia) and possibly a feeling of stiffness. You can relieve this by bending to the side and slightly turning the head. One may try to relieve the pain by bending the head in direction of the pain, because the discomfort is more tolerable in this position. Any divergence from this position causes immediate, intense pain.

Migraine-type headache may develop and cause nausea (cervical vertebral column migraine). Pain extends from the neck up to the temple as a tension headache.

Note: If the pain radiates via the shoulder into the arm and to the fingers, go see a doctor!

Causes

A "stiff neck" is frequently the consequence of extreme motion of the spine and fast turning of the head, for example in soccer, tennis, gymnastics, and golf. With a previously damaged spinal column, just one quick motion of the head can lead to acute pain. A draft through an open car window, especially with wet hair, is just as dangerous as a breeze coming from air conditioning in a car or room. A stiff neck may also be caused by a bed that is too hard or too soft, pillows that are too thick, as well as an unfamiliar sleeping position (turning or extending the head) in an airplane or bus. Moreover, the lop-sided carrying of luggage while traveling can lead to pain.

First Aid

For certain relief, Salonpas-hot "capsicum patch" cut to fit around the neck and shoulder region and applied carefully may work. Generally, it is tolerated by athletes in spite of the heat that it generates. Stroking the neck and shoulder areas can alleviate pain and increase relaxation. Rough massage, however, leads to increased pain.

Additionally, infra-red treatment (an infrared lamp) may be used. Cover the painful area with a warm, damp hand towel and heat the area with an infrared lamp for about 10-15 minutes from a distance of 16-20 inches. A gentle application of Marco Sport Blue or Green, Bengay, or "Born Again" salve reduces the pain.

Relieve pressure on the cervical spine by using a neck wrap: A rolled-up Turkish hand towel (3-4 inches wide) is loosely wrapped around the neck and fastened with two strips of tape.

The ideal support is created by filling a thin, elastic tricot stocking (such as Trico Fix, which is 3-4 inches wide and about 24 inches long) with reflective Rheumawadding, a wide bandage from the drugstore. Roll it to a length of 14-16 inches and a width of about 3-4 inches and insert into the stocking; leave both ends of the dressing with enough extra material to tie a knot. Place it around the neck and tie the ends of the stocking together.

Alternatively: Shape a hand towel into a firm, but not bulky, roll (2-3 inches diameter), fasten it with 3-4 strips of tape, and place it under the neck and relax on your back. Put a blanket roll beneath the knees. Perform gentle rolling motions of the head to the left and right from this position.

Hint: One can also obtain a comfortable and easy treatment from a good warm shower: Place a plastic or enamel stool or chair in the shower to sit on. Aim an increasingly warmer stream of water toward the shoulder and neck area. Simultaneously turn the head gently to the left and right to increase the range-of-motion. After that, dry the hair and skin well, but not roughly. Continue with measures to relieve discomfort, such as resting on the back with a neck-roll and bent knees. Gently let the head fall, allowing gravity to pull the head in both directions.

It is helpful to continue the therapy with warm Flexall or Cramergesic salve. Place a tube of the salve in hot water, then spread a half-inch thick application on a gauze compress that has been dampened with warm water. Have the patient lie down with the painful area on the compress. Cover the area with a large towel. The packing may be left on overnight.

Follow-Up Treatment

Stretching exercises for the neck are therapeutic. Have the athlete sit on a stool or chair, holding on to one side of the chair while bending the head in the opposite direction (until a mild pulling sensation occurs). Gently rotate the head. The exercises should be done 10-15 times, while alternating direction.

Another exercise recommendation: Have the athlete sit on a stool with the back straight and the head positioned over the body. Try with both hands to press the head forward against the firmly-tensed muscles of the neck. This is to be held for several seconds. Repeat the exercise 10-15 times. Mobilize the spinal column through treatments done by an experienced physical therapist. Exercises can then be repeated at home. If there is ongoing pain, go to see a doctor!

STRETCHING THE THROAT AND NECK MUSCULATURE:
The athlete sits on a stool and holds onto it with one hand, while the other hand clasps the head and pulls it to the side. Important: the shoulder of the opposite side must be held down in order to feel a pulling sensation. Duration: about 20 seconds.

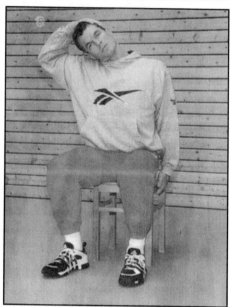

STRETCHING THE NECK MUSCULATURE:
The athlete sits on a stool with hands clasping the stool behind the back; the head is pressed forward with the chin upon the chest. Duration: about 20 seconds.

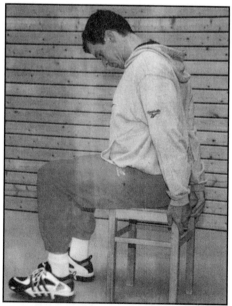

Prevention

Always perform a warm-up program, especially for the neck and shoulder areas (see "Practical Tips"), when racquet sports such as tennis, squash, or badminton are being played.

One should avoid jerky movements of the neck and shoulders before these areas are toned from warming up.

Blow your hair dry after the shower and avoid drafts, especially with wet skin and clothing. When perspiring heavily, be careful of wind or drafts; even with summer temperatures, skin and muscles can easily get chilled from heat loss due to evaporation. The muscles then tend to go in to spasm. Protect the neck area after a shower by placing a towel, shawl, or raised collar around it. Promptly exchange a wet shirt for a dry one.

Medications: Magnesium supplement each morning and evening, Vitamin E. (Consult your doctor.)

NOTES

All forms of Traumeel are available from:
Heel Inc.
1-800-621-7644

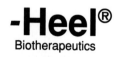

DISLOCATION OF THE SHOULDER

The dislocation of a shoulder is one of the most common joint injuries, especially in competitive sports involving ball playing, pitching, or tossing, as well as in skiing.

Dislocations are diagnosed when the end of the upper arm rolls from its joint cavity by being displaced forward, down, or back. Frequently, parts of the joint capsule and ligaments are ruptured. The shoulder cartilage can also be injured in the process.

Symptoms

Intense pain during motion and rest is experienced; the outline of the shoulder joint changes, as well as the placement of the arm. The patient holds the arm in a protective position because all movement causes pain.

Causes

A fall on an outstretched arm (such as during skiing, Judo, gymnastics, football, bicycling, or riding) — or an abnormal back-swing motion (typical in handball) are the most frequent causes of this injury.

First Aid

The patient must be promptly taken to a doctor's office or hospital, lying on his/her back if possible. No lay-person is equipped to try to adjust the shoulder. There may be a fracture of the upper arm.

Important: The arm needs a base of support (such as a sweater or a training jacket); it must not hang free. This is also taken into account by the paramedics who are transporting the athlete to the hospital.

Follow-Up Care

Care is directed by the doctor. A shoulder dislocation must be adjusted by a specialist as soon as possible. Generally, it will be kept immobile in a sling for about 3 weeks.

Prevention

Well-developed and trained muscles (in the shoulder area) are helpful in avoiding a dislocation. Some sports such as ice-hockey require special shoulder protection.

DISLOCATION OF THE CROMIOCLAVICULAR (A.C.) Joint

This joint connects the collar-bone and the shoulder-blade. It lies above the shoulder joint and is held by ligaments that get stretched and/or ruptured due to injuries.

Symptoms

Intense pain during movement, pressure, immobility, or rapid swelling. This shoulder injury cancels sports activities.

During the first month of recuperation, the arm hangs down as if paralyzed until the body instinctively and automatically bonds it to the upper body (the upper arm is generally held to the body in the "Napoleon posture"). The lower arm is placed on the chest. The hand usually grabs clothing for support. If ligaments have ruptured, we have the so-called "Piano-Key Syndrome": The clavicle (collar bone) is very loose and sticks up and out. It is the highest bone of the shoulder and can be pressed down like a piano key. Upon release, it resumes its prior position.

Causes

A dislocation of the A.C. joint usually occurs from an uncontrolled fall onto the shoulder from standing height, after a jump (during soccer, after running under a person in connection with a "header"), a pitch in handball, or after a body-check in ice-hockey.

First Aid

Cool with a "hot-ice" pressure bandage. Place an ice-water-saturated sponge (oval, about 2x4 inches in size, and a half-inch thick) on the injured area and wrap it tightly with an 3-4-inch wide Ace bandage. The bandage begins in the underarm area of the injured shoulder, includes the sponge and wraps around the shoulder joint. Continue to wrap over the chest and across the back to the other underarm until it is at the point of origin. Fasten the end of the bandage with two clips. Leave it in place for compression for about 20 minutes and repeat 4-5 times.

After first aid is completed, lay a piece of foam rubber, covered with Marco Sport Blue, X-Cell-R-Aid Salve or Neosporin ointment, on the injured area and secure it with a broad tape strip across the chest and back. A series of approximately 24-inch-long tape strips are then used, one after the other, to tape the preparation to the skin. The center of the tape strip sticks to the foam rubber and the tape reaches from the chest to the back. The tape should be tight and securely fastened. The ends of the vertically-running supports are connected by crosswise-running tape strips.

A more elaborate taping technique includes using the end of an Ace bandage. Affix it to the healthy shoulder as a harness. Pass it over the nape of the neck to the injured shoulder and the extended upper-arm. This covers the outside of the upper arm and is firmly taped in place.

Gravity automatically increases pressure on the arm and injured joint. For relief, the arm should be placed in a make-shift sling such as a shawl, binder, necktie, belt or piece of cloth.

The injured person must then be examined by a doctor.

Follow-Up Care

This is subject to the doctor's and the physical therapist's discretion.

Prevention

As with the dislocation of the shoulder: Good conditioning of the shoulder muscles and shoulder protectors for ice-hockey players are helpful.

SHOULDER STIFFNESS (bursitis)

The shoulder joint is the most movable joint of the body. Its superb anatomic construction is comprised of capsule, ligaments, muscles, and sinews which make the joint totally flexible. Even minor disturbances of these structures can lead to considerable difficulties, such as a stiff shoulder. One speaks of shoulder stiffness when the joint is inflamed and motion is extremely painful. This is caused by injury to the soft-tissue mantle (muscles, sinews, bursa, joint capsule).

Symptoms

When there is shoulder stiffness, severe pain often occurs in the upper-outer shoulder. It may cause total immobility. The injured person assumes a protective posture. The upper arm is instinctively pulled close to the body to protect the shoulder and to avoid additional pain. The patient gingerly lifts the arm. Raising of the arm occurs from the shoulder because of exquisite pain.

Lying on the affected side is also uncomfortable. Warmth from the shoulder area is rare.

Causes

Chronic over-stressing through use of one side of the body more than the other, or unfamiliar stress during extensive training exercises such as tennis serving or driving a golf ball are common causes. Trauma to the shoulder from a blow, fall, or kick may injure the joint, the ligament, sinews, muscles, or bursa. Wear and tear on the tendons and muscle attachments of the shoulder area, nerve root irritation of the lower neck or gout may be the culprits.

First Aid

Once injured, the shoulder joint needs careful use, not immobilization. Pain is reduced by hot showers. Expose the shoulder to a gentle stream of gradually increasing water temperature as a "massage". Subsequently, rub the area with a flat-sweeping motion. Use ice cube or ice on a stick (fill a small yogurt cup with water, place a tongue depressor or similar item into it and let it freeze). Apply this 3-4 times daily for 20 seconds, always drying the skin with a hand towel between treatments.

If localized heat from the shoulder is noticeable (compare both sides), an alcohol compress or a cold wrap will disperse the accumulation of heat. A compress is made with 70% rubbing alcohol, which is diluted with water to a ratio of 1:5. Saturate a small hand towel with the solution. Place it on the shoulder and cover with a dry towel. Do not use a plastic sheet in between! Repeat when the cooling effect begins to diminish. Alternatively, use a "hot-ice" bandage.

If the pain diminishes with the use of cold, a container of Flexall or Cramergesic salve can be placed in the refrigerator and used as a cold-pack.

If the pain is relieved by heat treatments, warm ointment in hot water and apply it as a warm pack. Spread the salve a half-inch thick on a dampened bandage roll or compress. Place it on the injured shoulder, and cover it with a dry hand towel and a binder. If possible, apply the packing for several hours.

We recommend motion exercises with the arm 2-3 times daily, in order to increase the pain-free zone. For instance, gentle swinging of the arm (forward and backward or to the side). Later, weight on the arm can be increased by holding a heavy object such as a book or bottle. Duration per exercise: 5-6 minutes.

Note: If acute pain occurs, or pain radiates to the lower arm via the elbow, promptly see a doctor. If the shoulder becomes stiff after a large meal or an alcoholic drink a doctor's examination is required. There may possibly be an elevated uric acid level (gout).

Medications: For the reduction of pain, take 3-6 tablets daily of Aspirin plus Vitamin C. (Consult your doctor.)

Follow-Up Care

It is recommended to do endurance exercises with the goal of restoring the original capacity of the joint. The guidance of an experienced physical therapist is absolutely necessary. Inactivity as well as protective immobilization quickly lead to adhesions (fibrous tissue deposits), the formation of callouses, and to shrinking of the shoulder joint capsule.

To avoid muscle weakness, training is recommended; this should be consistently practiced at home, after consultation with the physical therapist. Exercises for stretching, loosening, and strengthening are ideal (such as with an elastic band). The out-stretched arm pulls the band, which is fastened to a door handle, or other stationary object. Movement is directed forward, upward, and backward, while turning the out-stretched arm and bending the lower arm in and out.

Another very effective exercise, which can be done several times a day, includes the use of an elastic band affixed to the ceiling or a closet door. The out-stretched arm moves the band down and back simultaneously.

Important: Do the exercises consistently and cautiously. Stop if pain occurs.

Prevention

Take care to attain or maintain good muscle conditioning and develop the shoulder muscles. Avoid one-sided shoulder stress during training so that the muscle equilibrium is not disturbed.

Hint: For racquet sports do not neglect the opposite shoulder. It should receive special exercises. All of the muscles of the shoulder must undergo equal training. Avoid cold and drafts; do not ride in a car with an open window when you are perspiring. If your doctor advises you that your uric acid levels are elevated, use a low-protein diet as recommended by the doctor. Also, avoid alcohol.

NOTES

For more information about Marco Sport,
call Pro Nutrition at:
1-888-303-7668

"TENNIS ELBOW" / "GOLF ELBOW" / "PITCHER'S ELBOW"

Athletes label this common, painful injury "tennis elbow." This refers to an inflammatory condition originating in the tendons of the lower arm on the outside of the elbow, where the tendons are anchored to the bone. In its acute phase, "tennis elbow" causes intense pain, preventing any sports activities. The mere lifting of a cup of coffee, a glass, or even a gentle handshake, can be painful.

With timely and correct treatment, this can easily be remedied. If "tennis elbow" becomes chronic, however, healing may become long and difficult.

Acutely inflammatory "Tennis Elbow"

The type of pain associated with this condition is not easy to describe. It may arise suddenly after a difficult tennis match or after unfamiliar stress to one arm such as repeated twisting motions (turning a screwdriver), or it may develop gradually.

In the acute phase of this condition, intense pain will occur from clasping or lifting objects. Discomfort is felt on the outside elbow joint, which is pressure-sensitive. The pain center is often confined to a very limited area, but will sometimes radiate into the lower arm. It may cause stubborn muscle cramps below the elbow. Forget about playing tennis!

Hint: A simple test may reveal the presence of tennis elbow: Place the hand (palm down) on a table and try to raise the index finger and/or middle finger against resistance. Pain in the area of the elbow indicates "tennis elbow."

Golf Elbow and Pitcher's Elbow

An injury similar to tennis elbow often poses a problem for baseball pitchers, javelin throwers, and golfers. Complaints from these athletes occur on the *inside* of the elbow.

Causes

Pain arises from chronic irritation of the lower arm muscles and tendons through over-stress, or frequently from poor technique. For example, when the javelin is held too far from the body and too far back.

In golf, symptoms are also caused by over-stress (too much force instead of momentum at tee off), imperfect technique (deficient follow-through), and hitting the ground with the club. The treatment is identical to the treatment for "tennis elbow".

If pain fails to subside, a doctor must be consulted. "Tennis elbow" may represent an underlying condition of the elbow joint, including small ruptures within the joint ligaments, or, rarely, ruptured tendons.

First Aid

Special attention must be paid to avoiding conditions which cause discomfort — whether pain occurs at home or on the job. For example, the symptoms of "tennis elbow" often appear after hours of strenuous housework or repetitious work on a computer keyboard. Poor posture often leads to muscle dysfunction and, with that, back and neck discomfort. This promotes the development of "tennis elbow" and its related symptoms.

Until pain lessens, we recommend the application of multiple "hot-ice" bandages moistened with 2 Tbs. arnica tincture mixed with 1 pint of ice water, or a wet Ace bandage wrapped around the lower arm and elbow. Re-moisten the bandage from time to time. Inability to withstand cold at this stage could be a sign of a back problem. A visit to the doctor should be scheduled.

Alternatively, soak the arm in tepid water and, as a possible cure, add therapeutic oils, such as thyme or arnica to the water (submerge the elbow for 10-15 minutes); then rub the painful area with Marco Sport Blue.

A copper-quartz-rosemary tincture or Marco Sport Blue can be applied gently. This can be followed by the use of ointment-bandages (see "Practical Tips") which may be applied for several hours, using Marco Sport Blue, Betadine, and/or Traumeel Ointment or Flexall gel. Judiciously reapply the bandages every 8 hours.

Medications: Wobenzym, Magnesium supplements (consult your doctor for dosage),Vitamin E (400 mg: 2 cap. daily) and tablets of Aspirin + Vitamin C supplement over a period of 10 days.

Follow-Up Care
(see chronic "Tennis Elbow," below).

CHRONIC "TENNIS ELBOW"

Symptoms
"Chronic tennis elbow" develops after initial symptoms of the condition have been ignored. Unlike acute "tennis elbow," rest is not usually required for this condition. The pain is often steady and recurrent, thus complaints may last for weeks or months. Playing tennis is possible for limited periods of time, with a good partner or teacher who can do rhythmic playing for 45 minutes under suitable conditions. Include the use of an appropriate bandage. Only overextended play leads to renewed pain.

First Aid

Besides prescribed treatment from a physical therapist, damp heat is usually helpful. Place a damp hand towel over the elbow, cover it with plastic wrap, and apply a hot pack or heating pad for about 30 minutes. Ensure that the heat is maintained at a tolerable level. Turn the heating pad on and off to maintain an even temperature.

"Fire packing" (2x daily: 15-20 minutes) includes the use of a heat producing ointment. Spread thinly over the painful area. Extend treatment to the middle of the forearm and cover it with plastic wrap. Finally wrap it with a hot pack or heating pad.

Note: If a skin reaction should occur, remove the hot pack or heating pad immediately. Heat does not always alleviate pain. In some individuals, heat may create pain.

Subsequently, rub the affected area uniformly with ice (every 10-15 seconds, followed by 10-15 second pauses. Repeat 4-5 times).

Hint: Fill a small yogurt cup with water; place a tongue depressor or Popsicle stick into the cup and place it in the freezer. Later, one can apply the "Ice-on-a-Stick" to the uncomfortable area.

Follow-Up Care

As the acute condition subsides, stretching, strengthening and toning exercises to the lower arm area must follow. If symptoms continue, consult a physician.

Massage: Determine the painful areas with the thumb. Exert light pressure on the painful area and move the thumb from the inside to the outside, until the discomfort diminishes. Subsequently, massage the muscles surrounding the painful area across and up-and-down to the area of the elbow.

For the massage, we recommend the use of Marco Sport Blue or Green or Flexall gel.

Useful Exercises:

1. Stretching: Form a fist. Turn the hand inward so that the thumb points downward. Then stretch the elbow and push the arm outward. Angle the hand at the wrist far enough outward so that tension is felt in the muscles of the lower arm (repeat this exercise 5x, each time for 10-15 seconds).
2. Toning: Bend the elbow slightly and perform quick shaking motions with the hand. During this process, slowly raise the arm above the head.
3. Play tennis daily (without a ball) for a few minutes. Assume the correct stance. This is an opening position. Grip the racquet and use a back-swing motion. Use a full follow-through with the racquet.

Exercises for strengthening the extensor, flexor, and wrist muscles:

1. Opening position: Place the forearm on a table surface, while keeping the wrist at the table's edge. The hand should freely move up and down.
2. Muscle Stretching: Clasp the center of the tennis-racquet handle and slowly raise the arm to its maximal stretch. Then, relax the muscles of the arm slowly and bring the hand down again. Repeat 10 times until muscle fatigue is noticeable.
3. Bending Exercises: Repeat the previous exercise with the palm of the hand facing upwards.
4. Flexion Exercises: The palm should face downward as you

hold the racquet at a right angle in front of the body. The racquet is held so that its weight is evenly distributed across the palm. Now turn the hand in both directions; that is, to the left and to the right.

5. By holding the racquet near the handle grip or by practicing with small weights (maximum weight of 2 lbs), one can increase the effect of the training. However, because the effect of practice is measured by the level of muscle fatigue, maximum effect is possible by increasing the rate of exercise. Be sure to increase pauses between "reps" and as increased fatigue is felt.

Important for all exercises: Never train while in pain!

Causes and Prevention

Due to improved training techniques, as well as improved equipment, complaints of tennis elbow injuries have been reduced in recent years. However, over-exertion, improper equipment, and incorrect movements remain the most frequent causes of tennis elbow. To avoid this painful condition in the first place observe the following advice:

Preparation:

To avoid typical tennis injuries, good general health and active warm-up exercises are needed. The bad habit of going to the tennis court "cold" and immediately starting a match, is unfortunately very popular. It is correct and wise to warm up first. A brief run is ideal — enough to work up a mild sweat — then proceed with stretching exercises tailored to the thighs and back muscles, as well as the shoulders (see "Practical Tips").

At least 15 minutes of warm-up is necessary before the first serve in tennis. Golfers should allow 10 minutes of warm-up in order to properly loosen the back, shoulder, and arm muscles before the first swing.

Track and field runners need more than 60 minutes to reach the correct "motion temperature" for peak performance.

Hint: Rub a few drops of Marco Sport Red mixed with a few drops of thyme or arnica oil into the muscles of the neck and upper and lower arms before play or practice begins. Also, tennis elbow supports (such as Epitrain Bandage) may be temporarily applied. They help to reduce stress to the lower arm while "massaging" the area.

The Racquet:

The selection of a good racquet is extremely important. Consult a trainer or a tennis "pro" for advice before making the purchase. The modern, plastic racquets with broad frames and enlarged hitting surfaces absorb vibrations better than the older metallic racquets. However, bad decisions about racquet weight always remain a risk factor for the tennis player.

The Strings:

Amateur tennis players attempt to mimic the tennis "pros" by having their racquets strung too tightly, according to reports by the media. They mistakenly believe that extremely taut strings are the secret of success. In actuality, the tautness of the strings must be suited to the playing skills and body-type of each individual. Softer strings offer greater elasticity, and are therefore more forgiving when hitting the ball than tighter strings. Hard strings require absolute precision, since one must hit the ball dead-center. An off-center hit with hard strings exposes the athlete's lower arm to more intense vibration. This can cause damage to the lower arm and elbow later on.

The Handle:

The size of the handle must be correct. A handle that is too thick or too thin requires more strength and thereby increasing the danger of over-stressing a swinging arm. Anyone can determine the right handle size. Clasp the racquet handle loosely with the left hand. When the athlete can place the little finger of the other hand between the tip of the ring finger and the ball of the hand they have found a racquet that fits. Now and then, the hand grip should be replaced.

Striking Technique:

Frequently, the lower arm muscles become over-stressed through poor technique, such as too much exertion instead of using the ball's momentum. All beginners, youths, and "return" players are prone to doing this. Therefore, our advice is to start the game with a "clean" striking technique.

Use a full back-swing. Allow the stroke its full swing, do not break it prematurely. A poor follow-through is physiologically incorrect and is made at the expense of the tendons. A "back-hand-slice" and/or a "top-spin," for instance, require practice. Their mechanics are complex. Correctly executed, such moves are useful, but a poorly-executed "back-hand-slice" or "top-spin" is dangerous.

Balls:

Go for good quality when buying tennis balls. Do not use them too long. Be especially aware of wet or damp courts. When there is rain, the ball absorbs dampness, becomes heavier, and places excessive stress upon the arm muscles.

Tip: When returning to practice after a long absence, take a few lessons from an experienced instructor who can help you get back in the game with the most effective technique. If possible, check out your technique through video analysis. It is better to have too much training than too little!

Tennis Court Surfaces:

The tennis court surface — and the change from one type of surface to another — can lead to the development of tennis elbow. Clay courts, with their slightly slippery surfaces, allow for easier access to the ball and a more precise return. They are optimal in the prevention of tennis elbow.

On other surfaces, however, such as concrete, artificial turf, plastic, or carpet, the ball bounces faster. The motion of the ball becomes flatter. The spin is more difficult to calculate; and preparation time to reaching a ball is shorter. This chain of events often leads to errors in striking technique. Unplanned, chaotic movement results in the hand and lower arm attempting to balance the defective swing in a split-second, using jerky, cramped motions. The frequent result: "tennis elbow."

Stress:

Just like golf, tennis also has its share of "addicts." However, those who are new to the game, have not practiced, or those who play infrequently should be careful not to overdo. These enthusiasts need to remember that too much is unhealthy. It is recommended that these players arrange a 2-3 day pause between training sessions or games — to allow their bodies sufficient recovery time.

These are the usual reasons for the ailment called "tennis elbow." However, there are contributing causes, or additional factors, which are diagnosed by a doctor. Among these are unrecognized diseases including infected teeth, tonsils, and sinuses, prostate inflammation, elbow disturbances, low back problems and gout.

NOTES

For more information about Wobenzym call:
1-888-4-VITAMINS
(1-888-484-8264)

NOTES

For more information about Jurlique Call:
1-800-854-1110

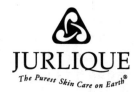

INJURIES OF THE FINGERS

Without the hand, its fingers, and their joints, most sports activities would be severely limited — the hand grabs firmly, hits, pushes, reaches, supports, presses, hurls, points, etc. The philosopher Aristotle once stated: "The hand is the instrument of instruments." The hand is a wonder of anatomical design. When it is injured, the average human — especially the athlete — is disabled in the truest sense of the word. The range of injuries is endless. Compression, strain, dislocation, ruptured and torn tendons, injuries to the joint capsule or joint-ligament apparatus, as well as chipped bones and fractures can occur during trauma.

Symptoms

Injuries to the fingers are disproportionately painful. The course of healing is often long and protracted. At times there is considerable pain due to motion and pressure. Usually, after just a short time, severe swelling will occur.

The injured finger may deviate from normal positioning. When alignment is lost, there is a feeling of joint instability. When there is a rupture of an extensor muscle (those which return the hand to a normal position), the fingers can no longer be bent at an angle. When symptoms include either intense pain, severe swelling, instability, or abnormal appearance, a medical examination and care are required.

Causes

A fall with splayed fingers or a blow are frequently the cause of finger trauma. Finger injuries may occur after a ball hits the finger tips. Especially vulnerable are goalkeepers (handball, soccer), as well as volleyball and basketball players.

Additional causes include getting the hand caught on the uniform of another player, or a glancing blow to the hand from a ball or shot-put. "Skier's-thumb" is an injury which frequently occurs after catching a gloved thumb within the grip of a ski-pole. As with the condition known as "baseball-finger" (ruptured finger tendons), a diagnosis from an ER doctor and appropriate treatment, possibly including surgery, is necessary.

First Aid

For mild "jammed fingers" and dislocations, non-professional help is adequate. Wrap a "hot-ice" pressure bandage (see "Practical Tips") with an ice-water saturated small sponge or cloth inside it. A good choice for a bandage is 1-3/4 inch Gazofix wrapped around the entire finger — not just a part of it, as circulatory disturbances may result from partial bandaging. Wet the bandage periodically using ice water. Loosen the pressure bandage after 20 minutes, then re-apply it after about a two-minute pause (repeat 3-4 times).

In case of a serious injury, do not apply a pressure bandage. Use only a Gazofix bandage, or cotton towel, saturated with ice water and wrapped around the injured joint. In the case of "skier's-thumb," the injured finger should be splinted to the next finger. To do this, lay a piece of foam rubber between the fingers. Bend the fingers slightly and wrap them in gauze. Change the bandage daily for the next 10 days, or as needed.

Medications: Until the symptoms diminish, the intake of either Traumeel tablets or Wobenzym (consult your doctor for correct dosages) is recommended. The application of ice, pressure, and ointment-bandages are also advisable.

Injuries of the joints or ligaments require gentle care and careful positioning. In addition to using the fingers as splints, (which is suitable for injuries of the fingertips) there are the ready-made finger splints available in many sizes for adults and children. They cover the finger joints and may be worn for weeks. Generally, some sports activity is possible with these. To deal with a finger injury most effectively, it is always best to obtain an X-ray as a precaution. Unfortunately, fractures and ruptures frequently get overlooked.

Follow-Up Care

When there is a noticeable muscle weakness of the hand, the muscles of the hand and fingers should be strengthened through exercises with either a softball, therapeutic kneading material, rubber ball, light weight, and/or a short interval before returning to sports activities.

Prevention

In many sports, injuries to the finger(s) can be prevented (especially skiing, snow-boarding, ice-skating, ice-hockey, or skateboarding) by always wearing special gloves. However, volleyball players, basketball players, shot-putters, and goalkeepers, are advised to "tape" the finger joints with tape strips. This especially makes sense when there have been previous injuries. Athletes who are frequently exposed to hand injuries are encouraged to perform loose finger exercises, as well as special strength training for fingers and hands.

FRACTURED SCAPHOID (wrist) BONE

An injury to the fleshy part of the thumb is often labeled a joint compression. This frequently-overlooked fracture of the scaphoid bone is usually caused by a fall on the hand when it is outstretched, or from a ball slamming against the palm of a goalkeeper. Misdiagnosis and mistreatment of a fractured scaphoid can lead to disability later on. A doctor's examination is required.

Symptoms

Localized pain, sensitivity to pressure, pain with movement, swelling and internal bleeding (with the hand sometimes appearing bluish), as well as weakness of the thumb are all common.

First Aid

Until medical examination and treatment take place, swelling and bruising must be minimized. Cool with "hot-ice" (see "Practical Tips").

Important: If an X-ray examination is inconclusive, we recommend tomography (CAT Scan) or, after 8-9 days, an X-ray series. Sometimes, the X-rays fail to clearly indicate a fracture until a full week passes.

Therapy: Long-term immobilization with a cast (three to four months) is usually called for, followed by an intensive program of rehabilitation by a physical therapist. If the fracture is badly displaced — depending on the extent — surgery (Osteosynthesis) can promote safer and faster healing.

Serious athletes have a tendency to prefer surgical care. We recommend acquainting oneself with the name of a hand surgeon if regular activities involve any risk to the hands.

NOTES

Hastings House Book Publishers
Tel: 203-838-4083
Fax: 203-838-4084

HASTINGS HOUSE

NOTES

All forms of Traumeel are available from:
Heel Inc.
1-800-621-7644

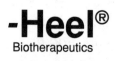

LOCAL WOUNDS / NOSE-BLEEDS

Tears and local wounds to the head often appear more dramatic and serious than they are due to the presence of heavy bleeding. Bleeding is unusually heavy because the skin of the head is well supplied with blood vessels. Local wounds over a half-inch in length must be promptly treated by a doctor who will usually "stitch up" the wound. If the patient appears confused or dazed, there is danger of concussion (bleeding inside the head).

Symptoms

Usually, very heavy bleeding is present from the eyebrows, nose, chin or the scalp.

Causes

Injuries to the head usually occur through violent impact — such as a hit, thrust, or kick — and they   require immediate professional treatment.

First Aid (Localized Small Wounds)

Small local wounds: Dab the injured area with peroxide and apply pressure with a sterile gauze compress. Place a small, sterile cotton bandage on the bleeding area and tape firmly with a large band-aid. When bleeding stops, and if the patient has no dizziness, activity can usually resume.

> **Note:** Keep the injured area dry during a shower; do not wash it! After a shower the wound can be disinfected with a sterile cotton swab and a new bandage can be applied.

Large local wounds: Wounds larger than a half-inch in length must be sutured or stapled by a doctor. Keep the wound clean and completely covered by a sterile cotton dressing; affix it with a large band-aid or tape. Finally, clean the area surrounding the wound, so that the extent of the injury can be evaluated. Apply pressure to stop bleeding. See a doctor as fast as possible!

Important: Check out Tetanus immunization records.

Prevention

Exposed areas of the face should be covered with a thin film of Vaseline before any sports activity. Boxers and athletes in other competitive sports would do well to apply some Vaseline to the eyebrows, chin, cheeks and nostrils.

First Aid (Nosebleeds)

Clean the face with a sponge. Then, apply a rolled gauze compress in the affected nostril until the bleeding stops. Press the nostrils firmly together. Generally, the sports activity may be continued unless bleeding continues. If unable to stop bleeding, see a doctor.

CONCUSSION (Commotio cerebri)

If there is the slightest suspicion of a concussion after an accident, the activity must immediately be stopped and a doctor must be seen. There is no playing-around with a concussion. It is a serious injury.

Symptoms

Failing memory: Usually, the injured athlete is unable to remember events relating to the accident. They cannot recall the exact sequence. The patient may be dazed over a period of time, but will usually possess a rough idea about where they are and what time it is (after the initial dizziness subsides). However details of the accident elude them because there is no recall. The patient is not aware of the circumstances surrounding the accident in the case of a brain concussion.

"What has happened?" If the injured athlete can provide no information to this concrete question, one must assume that a concussion has occurred. However, loss of memory may also apply to the time preceding or following the accident (retrograde/anterograde amnesia). In other words, the injured athlete may remember the accident, but has no memory about what happened afterwards.

Balancing problems and dizziness: The injured athlete appears pale, very dazed, and in many cases has balancing problems — the patient can hardly stand up without assistance. Additionally, they may vomit or feel nauseous, as well as suffer from a headache and weakness.

Blood pressure: Pulse rate and blood pressure will decline in the event of a brain concussion.

Note: Bleeding or secretion of a clear fluid from either the mouth, nose, or ears, is indicative of a possible fracture at the base of the skull. These symptoms may also signal the occurrence of a potentially fatal case of brain bleeding. When the slightest suspicion of such an injury arises, a CAT Scan, X-ray, or MRI will be ordered by a physician. Transport the patient immediately to a hospital for examination and treatment. If possible, call 911.

Causes

Violent impact to the head, such as a collision, fall, blow, or kick may produce severe head injuries.

First Aid

It is extremely important that the first-aid provider remain calm and provide a clear, open space around the injured athlete. Speak calmly to the patient, and if possible, do basic first aid to the wound. Ask the patient to recall the course of the accident.

The presence of a brain contusion or cerebral hemorrhage (bleeding) can be established, among other ways, by testing the pupils. They will display a loss of reaction to light. The left and right pupils will react differently to the following two tests (evaluation has to be performed by a doctor, nurse or paramedic):

Index finger test: Move the index finger back and forth at a slow speed before the eyes of the injured athlete. The pupils must be able to follow the movements.

Light test: The eyes should react to a beam of light directed at the pupils by equal constriction (growing smaller) of the left and right pupils, individually.

Additional Test: Place a hand over the eye of the injured athlete. Since the pupil of the eye widens in the dark, the removal of the hand should cause the pupil to constrict.

In the event of a brain concussion, brain contusion, or cerebral hemorrhage, or when the slightest suspicion arises as to the state of the injured, a doctor should be seen immediately. The injured athlete should never be allowed to continue playing.

Overzealousness is inappropriate at this time. Permanent damage may occur. Life is threatened.

During transport to the hospital, raise the upper body of the injured athlete into a slightly sitting position. Apply warm blankets, and keep the patient under observation. Listen for regular breathing. The anxiety he or she may feel at this time may lead to hyperventilation. In this situation, calming words are helpful. Try to sympathetically encourage the patient to breathe slower. If the patient is nauseous, position on the side (to prevent choking on the vomit).

Caution: Twenty-four to forty-eight hours after the accident, the condition of the patient may deteriorate due to the presence of bleeding in the head (subdural hematoma).

If fainting occurs: Stay calm! The forehead and nape of the neck of the injured athlete should be covered with cold, damp hand towels, the legs should be elevated and the injured party's blood pressure taken.

Important: Even if the patient's condition improves, do not try to give food, drink, or medications — until a doctor has diagnosed the problem and authorized oral intake.

Follow-Up Care

Further treatment should be provided by a doctor who also must decide when sports activity may be resumed. With a brain concussion, count on a 2-3 week recuperation. Patience is required! Otherwise, long-term damage may result, as in continuing susceptibility to headaches or more serious problems.

Prevention

Never embark upon risk-laden sports activities when in poor physical condition. During "risky" sports activities such as ice-hockey, sledding and bobsledding, the use of protective helmets should be mandatory. This is also advised for cyclists and skiers.

NOTES

For more information about Marco Sport,
call Pro Nutrition at:
1-888-303-7668

NOTES

For more information about Wobenzym call:
1-888-4-VITAMINS
(1-888-484-8264)

Wobenzym®

FRACTURES

A fracture usually results in a forced rest for the athlete. It may last several weeks. When a bone's elasticity is overstressed, a fracture occurs. It is frequently connected with severe symptoms, such as intense pain and considerable inability to function. By contrast, stress fractures are hardly noticed by the injured athlete and are often misinterpreted as a contusion, or inflammation. Any exercise on a fractured bone can take place only after the healing process is completed (callus formation).

Upon suspicion of a fracture, immediate transport to the doctor is required. If there is any doubt about how to proceed in the case of serious injury, promptly call an ambulance or 911.

Symptoms

A fracture is often recognized by a clicking or grating sound. It usually corresponds with considerable loss of mobility, including total incapacity or abnormal movement of the injured limb. A change in the limb's appearance and rapid swelling usually indicate a fracture. As a rule, a fracture is accompanied by intense pain and comparatively heavy bleeding. Pain is especially noticeable in the case of fractured fingers or toes, or in the area of the knuckles or thighs. In contrast, fractured ribs usually elicit fewer complaints.

Heavy bleeding, numbness, or a strong localized tingling sensation point to a simultaneous injury of larger blood vessels or nerves. Weakness, nausea and shock from blood loss are the most significant secondary symptoms.

In a "compound fracture," skin and tissue surrounding the fracture are injured and the fractured bones are exposed.

Causes

A fracture is usually caused by a violent accident, such as a fall, shove, kick, or blow. However, fractures caused by stress following intensive and ongoing compression, such as of the lower thighs, may occur independently of violent outside effects. They usually appear as an injury to the tissue surrounding the bone (periostitis) that becomes visible only after a complete series of X-rays has been taken. Fractures resulting from one's own activities, such as the upper arm fracture of a javelin thrower, are rarer. They are sometimes brought about by calcium deficiencies, among other causes.

First Aid

If you suspect a possible fracture of the foot, knuckles, or any other bone, do not ignore it! Do not leave the scene of the accident until aid is provided, and never place any stress on the injured area!

Anyone assisting in the transport of the patient must use great caution. It is recommended that several people become involved, particularly in cases where a stretcher is needed (upon which the injured must be secured with a belt). If the patient has fainted or if there is any suspicion of injury to the spinal column, transport of the injured must be performed exclusively by trained professionals (an emergency medical technician or paramedic). The threat of paralysis or damage to the spinal cord is always present whenever there is a spinal column fracture.

Important: Never change the position of the patient when there is a suspected injury to the spinal column. Call for emergency assistance!

To avoid any danger of choking (blockage of the breathing paths by vomit or other obstruction of the windpipe), lay the patient on his/her side. In case of circulatory problems (low blood pressure), raise the legs of the injured party above the level of the heart. Place a damp hand towel on the forehead and nape of the neck; and ensure shade or sufficient heat (cover the patient with a blanket or jacket if appropriate). Fresh air is needed, also. Never leave the injured party alone. He/she should not eat or drink until a doctor's examination is performed. No pain-killers should be administered: Surgery may be delayed as a result of it.

In the case of a compound fracture — as long as the injured is still conscious — care of the wound with a topical solution such as peroxide is allowed. Cover the wound with sterile cotton compresses and loosely wrap it with a bandage (such as a flexible-stretch bandage). Never attempt to treat a fracture with an ice bag! Never place a pressure bandage, or any type of elastic bandage on the fracture. A fracture should be left alone as much as possible.

If abnormal position changes are evident in the bones of the limbs, e.g., an interrupted shin or a distorted ankle joint, no bandage — not even a light covering, should be placed on it until after the arrival of the ambulance.

For fractures of the foot, or arm bones, remove all pressure from the area. Attend to any abrasions or bleeding, and use a splint (if necessary, improvise!), for example place ski poles, on each side of the injured body part, and tie them loosely together, omitting the immediate area of the fracture. Depending on the area of the fracture, the splint should support joints located above and below the break, such as the hand and the elbow, or the ankle and the knee. Position the injured body part as high as possible. Promptly locate a doctor.

Follow-Up Care

Further treatment depends on the evaluation of the attending physician.

Prevention

Protect vulnerable body parts with padding (gloves, bandages, knuckle and tibial protection). If there is a history of previous injuries, tape the fingers before sports events (handball, volleyball, basketball, shot-put). Maintain good general health as well as a daily, well-planned training schedule (see "Practical Tips"). The improved coordination and body control that results will lower the threat of injuries.

NOTES

For more information about Jurlique Call:
1-800-854-1110

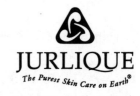

NOTES

Hastings House Book Publishers
Tel: 203-838-4083
Fax: 203-838-4084

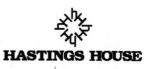

HASTINGS HOUSE

LACERATIONS AND SMALL CUTS

Due to their tendency to bleed heavily, such wounds often appear more serious and dramatic than they actually are. With expert and thorough care, these injuries usually heal very fast and without complications. Generally, wounds more than 1/2 inch long must be treated by a physician. For smaller injuries, non-professional care is fine.

Symptoms

May include heavy bleeding which can be quickly stopped.

Causes

Violent causes include effects from a kick, blow, shove, or fall.

First Aid

Clean the surrounding skin with a clean, wet cloth, then disinfect the tear or wound with Betadine (never use iodine or full-strength alcohol). After about 2-3 minutes, wipe the wounded area with a sterile compress. When there is considerable dirt in the wound, apply hydrogen-peroxide (3%) to the injured area. Its bubbling, foaming action rinses out dirt particles from the wound. To stop subsequent bleeding, use gauze bandages or butterfly sutures placed over the wound.

If these substances are not at hand, rinse the soiled wound or cut with clean water and disinfect with tea tree oil as quickly as possible. A shower should never be taken, because the dirt may get rinsed deeper into the wound. The wounded area, after cleansing, gets patted dry, covered with a sterile cotton compress, and wrapped up with an elastic bandage. Do not use any type of bandage with cotton fibers which will get caught in the wound, thereby increasing the probability of an infection.

Gaping wounds should be repaired with stitches and covered

by a sterile compress. Then they should be wrapped with an Ace bandage, or similar, in wide widths and at moderate tension. (A physician or physician's assistant should perform this treatment in a minor ER)

> **Important**: If the length of the cut or the laceration is more than 1/2 inch, a doctor should promptly be sought. They will make the decision about further treatment (such as staples or suturing). Ugly scars (keloids) may develop from incompetent treatment. Check the immunization record for a current Tetanus inoculation.

Follow-Up Care

Large wounds should receive on-going treatment by a physician who will also make the decision about when to resume sports activity. The date of return depends on the extent of the injury and its course of healing.

Prevention

Protect exposed body parts when involved in "risky" sports activities. Use shin guards (soccer, rollerblading), gloves (skiing, skateboarding, mountain-biking,) helmets (cycling).

ABRASIONS (scrapes)

Such injuries of the skin are among the most frequent sports accidents. They are often seen as "small stuff" and not taken seriously. However, when skin gets shaved off, there is always a danger of bacterial infection.

Careful treatment is required, otherwise, a severe inflammation and subsequent infection may develop in the wounded area. The adjoining lymph nodes (glands) may also swell up and cause pain.

Symptoms

Abrasions often make themselves known by a burning pain that is generally accompanied by mild or barely visible bleeding.

Causes

Skin abrasions are generally caused by a fall on a hard surface (halls or asphalt), artificial turf, or icy ground.

First Aid

Through immediate disinfection of the wound area with peroxide or tea tree oil, bacteria are killed and an inflammation is prevented. If the surrounding uninjured skin areas are dirty, clean the area with an alcohol wipe. Spray the wound itself with Bactine or run tap water over it to allow any dirt particles to be rinsed from the wound. As with the treatment of deeper wounds, take care not to force embedded dirt in deeper with a sponge, cloth, or strong water pressure. Pour diluted hydrogen peroxide (3%) over the wound for a rinse, (the foaming action of the hydrogen peroxide will loosen the dirt particles). Subsequently, gently pat the affected area with gauze 4x4's that are saturated with hydrogen peroxide.

The pink-appearing skin should then be disinfected again with an antibacterial ointment. To avoid complications in the healing process of the wound, it is recommended that any excess hair around the laceration be removed with a disposable razor.

Follow-Up Care

Cover the wound with a sterile compress such as Actisorb Plus by Johnson & Johnson. This is applied with a sticky flexible bandage or an extra large size band-aid. This type of protective care is helpful when treating certain locations on the body, such as the upper thigh, where a cumbersome bandage is often superfluous.

Tip: It is recommended that the wound be left open to the air as much as possible to enable drying. To achieve this, a fan can be used. Place it at a reasonable distance from the affected area, blowing mild warm air over the wound. Use a disinfectant before drying. If the wound should come in contact with fabric, it should be re-bandaged, as described. Fabric often causes friction and irritation which blocks the formation of scabbing.

Important: Make sure that Tetanus protection is up-to-date; if in doubt, check with your doctor. If no inflammation develops, the sports activity may be resumed after appropriate care of the injured area. If there is reddening or swelling of the wounded area, accompanied by a fever and enlargement of the lymph nodes (glands) of the groin or underarm, a doctor should be seen immediately. They will proceed with the necessary treatment and recommend resumption of any sports activities at the proper time.

Prevention

Protect the skin from abrasions by wearing long tights or training pants, especially in winter. Use of Lycra "biker's pants" for the game of soccer has successfully led to fewer abrasions in that sport, especially of the upper thigh. Falls resulting in skin abrasions occur not only on hard surfaces, but also on lawns covered by sand. Goalkeepers should make it a rule to wear special padded clothes and gloves to protect their knees and elbows, whether they are outside (especially on hard surfaces) or inside a stadium.

Tip: Cover vulnerable areas with Vaseline or baby oil.

NOTES

All forms of Traumeel are available from:
Heel Inc.
1-800-621-7644

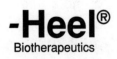

NOTES

For more information about Marco Sport,
call Pro Nutrition at:
1-888-303-7668

INFLAMMATION OF A TENDON OR TENDON SHEATH

Inflammation of the tendon, or the synovial sheath, can be extremely painful. If treatment is delayed, insufficient, or if the athlete fails to protect the affected area of the hand or ankle joint, there is a danger of a chronic condition that may require a lengthy recuperation period, and immobility. Prompt medical treatment is required.

Symptoms

Considerable pressure along with intense pain with motion and swelling in the affected area are symptomatic. Complaints occur in the area of the ankle, especially in the morning after getting up. Relief occurs with motion, sometimes after only a few steps.

In case of an acute inflammation of a tendon/synovial sheath, the injured athlete notices a crunching noise during motion, similar to the sound made when forming a snowball. For example, if one holds the Achilles tendon between thumb and index finger while moving the foot up and down, this "grinding" is easily felt. Pressure from either bandages or palpation can cause or intensify pain.

Causes of inflammation in the ankle joint area: Direct trauma such as a kick or blow from an opponent's shoe or tight shoes. An irritation of the tendon-sheath can also be caused by a bruise or scar formation. Pressure leads to a narrowing of the tendon canal, causing a rubbing on the tendon, and with it inflammation. A physical abnormality, for example flat-feet, may also lead to complaints.

Causes in the area of the hand joint: An inflammation of the tendon sheath of the hand is usually caused by stress during training, competition, or repetitive motions against resistance (such as during rowing or power-training). It can also come from improper or unfamiliar exercises.

First Aid

With the first appearance of discomfort, one should begin consistent cooling of the painful area, using "hot-ice" (made with 2 Tbs. arnica tincture blended with one quart of ice water). Saturate a cotton compress or a hand towel with the solution and wrap loosely with an Ace bandage (3 inches wide), using minimal pressure. Be careful that no folding or compressing of the skin occurs from wrapping the bandage.

When the cold effect diminishes, replace the "hot-ice" bandage or add plain ice water. The cooling may be continued for 8 hours. Full rest and care is mandatory during the acute phase!

At night, apply an ointment-bandage. Spread arnica gel or arnica cream on the affected area first, then apply an absorbent compress spread with a thick paste of ointment: Marco Sport Blue or Traumeel ointment, Neosporin, Cramergesic, or Flexal ointment are recommended.

Medications: To assist the healing process, the following medications are recommended: Bromalin capsules, Wobenzym, or Traumeel tablets. Take aspirin and vitamin C for pain relief. (Consult your doctor for required dosage.)

Immobilization

In very acute cases, when it is uncertain whether the tendon has been injured, provide temporary immobilization through a removable splint, or a pre-packed support bandage for the ankle.

Any long-term immobilization leads to increased weakness of the affected muscles. This is especially undesirable in this case. A cast has the disadvantage of blocking treatment, such as "hot-ice" applications.

Follow-Up Care

To help acute symptoms subside, follow-up care by a physical therapist is recommended. Also suggested are application of an anti-inflammatory ointment or gel, such as Bengay or Tiger Balm.

After acute pain subsides, muscle support and convalescent exercises should be used to strengthen the affected muscles (tendon and muscles work as a unit).

Later, we recommend exercising on your own to train the muscles of the lower arm or lower leg with elastic bands (for example Physiobands), arm or leg weights, or light weights.

Important: Avoid repetition of the muscle stress which led to the original problem. With correct and consistent treatment, tendonitis subsides after 7-10 days. In chronic cases, the injury may remain for several months.

Prevention

Do not undertake premature or intensive training after the injury heals. A general toning of the muscles appreciably lowers the risk of a relapse.

Provide routine attention to the care of the muscles, including stretching and loosening of the vulnerable areas, both before and after training or any competition. Use care when you bandage the hands and knuckles. Excess tightening of the tendon sheaths causes irritation which may lead to tendonitis.

If there is misalignment in the foot area — especially in the rear part of the foot — or ankle rotation — an orthotic is needed.

BURSITIS

Soccer goalkeepers and basketball, volleyball, and handball players complain of cases of bursitis due to their frequent falls. Usually, these occur in the area of the elbow, hip, and knee. The synovial bursae, lying between skin and bones, or between tendons and bones, serve a protective function for the tendons and, simultaneously, to decrease a hit or pressure on the structures close to the joint. If inflammation develops through a hit, kick, or pressure, it must be treated by a doctor immediately.

Bursitis requires gentle care until it is fully healed. This injury cannot "tolerate" any kind of pressure; therefore, proceed carefully when applying any kind of bandage! If the bursitis fails to be recognized and treated, the healing process may take weeks or months. In the case of therapy resistance, surgery may be required. However, if one understands the danger and undertakes the prompt treatment, complaints usually subside after only 2-3 days. In case of a fever or severe swelling, a doctor should be consulted immediately.

Symptoms

Acute pain due to pressure and motion, with usually clearly visible and palpable swelling and heat, are common. Characteristic of bursitis is a crunching sensation felt under the skin (like when one shapes a snowball) while touching or moving the skin at the point of discomfort. In acute cases, swelling may develop, along with reddening and heat.

Causes

Bursitis inflammation develops due to kicks, blows, or shoves. However, ongoing pressure from tight shoes, inflammation from the seams of a shoe, or at the heel, infections (e.g. after skin injuries), or gout can also cause or be contributing factors.

First Aid

Initially even the smallest skin wound must be treated due to the danger of infection. The location of injury (knee and elbow areas are especially vulnerable) is to be disinfected with peroxide, Mercurochrome or tea tree oil. If no disinfectant is at hand, clean the wound with fresh running water (without a forceful stream!). Never wipe the wound with a sponge, cloth or hand towel. Finally, cover the wound with a sterile compress.

Note: Direct pressure to the arm should be somewhat milder than in the legs; otherwise there is danger of swelling of the hand and fingers. Compression should not be applied for 20 minutes — as is recommended for other injuries — but for only 10 minutes. However, several repetitions of the compression are acceptable.

To prevent a swelling, sit or lie down after applying the compression bandage. Do not allow the affected extremity (arm or leg) to hang down. Position it above the level of the heart.

Should inflammation develop, visit a doctor, who may possibly need to drain the area. This is especially recommended when there is heavy bleeding in the joint spaces bursae; otherwise, clots remain. This may cause ongoing sensitivity and new inflammation.

Follow-Up Care

If the skin remains uninjured, apply an ointment-bandage with Marco Sport Blue ointment, or a healing earth (Luvos Healing Earth pack) for the night.

For open wounds use ointments which cause no irritation to the tissues, e.g. Traumeel ointment. Spread thickly on damp cotton gauze and apply with a damp, cold Ace bandage. Never wrap healing-earth packs or bandages in plastic. This may block the release of heat.

Medications: Beside Aspirin and Vitamin C, take Wobenzym or Bromalin capsules and Traumeel or AB drops #11. (Consult your doctor for individual dosage.)

For all cases of bursitis, resume training only after complete healing has taken place. Avoid pressure from clothing, bandages, or shoes. Also avoid heat applications due to the danger of causing inflammatory reactions.

Prevention

Wear protective bandages and padding for training and competition if areas are vulnerable. Goalkeepers should generally wear elbow protectors.

> **Tip #1:** Amateur and part-time goalkeepers should, like the "pros", wear padded pants (with increased hip protection) and knee protectors (especially on hard surfaces in the winter).
>
> **Tip #2:** If inflammation develops from rubbing against an inner shoe seam (at the joint behind the large toe or in the area of the heel), stretch the shoe in these areas. Spray the irritating spot with leather softener (Shu-eze). Then, insert shoe-trees or rolled up newspaper and leave in overnight.

NOTES

For more information about Wobenzym call:
1-888-4-VITAMINS
(1-888-484-8264)

Wobenzym®

NOTES

For more information about Jurlique Call:
1-800-854-1110

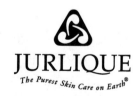

GROOMING AND HYGIENE

The normal standards for body grooming and hygiene should, naturally, apply in sports. Nevertheless, we would like to make some observations and offer some recommendations.

Bathing / Grooming

Showers or baths should be mandatory after training or competition. Because soaps disturb the protective coating of the skin (and an active athlete often needs to clean up repeatedly during the course of a day), it is advisable to use soap, shower gel, and shampoo sparingly; or rehydrating products should be used (such as ph5 Eucerin Lotion Soap and ph5 Eucerin shampoo).

After taking a shower, thoroughly dry the entire body with your own fresh towel. Blow-dry your hair. Even in warm weather there is danger of becoming over-chilled. This can result in a stiff neck. Do not merely groom the visible body parts, such as the fingernails, but also pay attention to toenails which also deserve regular cleaning and care.

Foot Care

Never go barefoot in the shower room or locker room, due to the danger of athlete's foot. Always wear your own bathing sandals or thongs; do not lend them. If an athlete already has a fungal disease (usually a foot fungus), the consistent application of either Athlete's Foot powder or spray is recommended and should include the spaces between the toes, socks, and the inside of the shoes. If there is a tendency towards sweaty feet, thoroughly dry them, then dry the spaces between the toes with a hair dryer, and treat with a suitable foot powder. Foot baths, followed by a pedicure and foot massage, improve one's feeling of general well-being.

To avoid the formation of blisters, rub the feet with Vaseline before extended training, jogging or stress due to hard floors.

Clothing

Use fresh underwear and fresh socks daily. Never leave wet towels and sports clothing in the gym bag, as they promote bacterial growth.

FUNCTIONAL OUTFITS AND CLOTHING

Shoes

For most sports activities, the shoe is the most important piece of equipment. With every jump, a sports shoe must absorb tremendous body weight. The shoe should cushion this effect, facilitate a smooth rolling step, stabilize, lead, and possibly compensate for orthopedic misalignments. Generally, only well known brands fulfill these requirements. The carefully selected shoe is the first step to avoiding injuries.

The variety of athletic footwear is plentiful. New and improved models are constantly reaching the market. Keep your footwear new and up-to-date.

When making a purchase: Check shoes for good workmanship. Athletic footwear bought on sale is often not worth it. It may actually turn out to be too expensive — because of later consequences to the feet and joints. Therefore, it is advisable to speak with a skilled specialist such as an orthopedist or athletic trainer when buying new athletic shoes. If possible, describe any difficulties you have experienced in the past; bring inlays or orthotics, or your old shoes along.

> **Tip:** It is advisable to bring your old, worn-out athletic shoes to the orthopedist when there are foot problems. For an expert, the run-down sole is perfect documentation of existing maladjustment from foot stress.

It is best to buy your shoes in the afternoon as size of the feet vary throughout the day from swelling. To avoid possible surprises from ill-fitting shoes, purchase athletic shoes only after sports activity. During the fitting, always try on both shoes and wear socks or stockings identical to those worn for the intended activity.

> **Tip:** If the athletic shoe is too small, tight, or irritating at a seam, spray these areas of the shoe with a leather-softener and stretch the shoe on a shoe tree overnight. Professional soccer players customarily wet their new shoes and then break them in.

Socks

To avoid blisters on sweaty feet, purchase only well-fitting socks which cannot bunch together. They should be made of cotton and have reinforced heels and toes.

Sports Clothes

Sports clothes, including shirts and shorts, are available in a variety of styles and fabrics. For training, a generously cut outfit, consisting of a cotton T-shirt and exercise shorts of synthetic/cotton blend, are ideal. Pure cotton fabric stays damp and absorbs about 20 times more water than synthetic fabrics such as polyester. Whenever possible, select cotton/polyester blends.

Net shirts allow air to pass through to the body and are

therefore recommended, especially in the summer. Perspiration has a chance to evaporate and the textile does not stick to the skin. Make sure before you buy them that shirts are very generously cut so that they do not chafe or irritate the skin. The same goes for shorts, which can cause irritation to the upper thighs due to sweating. The application of Vaseline to the skin provides protection.

> **Tip:** Wearing a pair of bicycle pants underneath your normal shorts is an effective way to prevent chafing and skin rashes, especially in the case of bicyclists or soccer players.

Beware of cold and drafts: Many athletes fail to pay attention to the weather. Even in warm temperatures, there is a danger of illness and discomfort (for example, stiffness of the neck) from excessive sweating followed by rapid evaporation. Tennis players should wear a sweater or a training jacket when practicing in the open air. This will keep the back warm until a proper "functional temperature" is maintained. This also applies when tennis players change sides, take breaks, or play on shady courts. In cold weather, a sweater, sweatshirt or even a training jacket is appropriate.

NUTRITION AND DRINKS

Good nutrition is an important condition for optimal performance in sports. Pay special attention to the intake of fluids before, during, and after training and competition. The athlete should expect a significant loss of perspiration, minerals and energy. According to our experience, considerable miscalculations are often made in this area.

Beverages

Training or competition lasting over an hour requires the replacement of lost body fluids and minerals during a break or at half time, especially in warm weather. When physical exertion goes on for several hours (as in tournaments), an athlete can lose 2-3 quarts of fluid, and sometimes even more. As little as 2% water loss leads to diminished performance!

For this reason, dehydration must be avoided with energy-rich mineral drinks. These can be consumed in small quantities during training, as well as during competitions. Lightly sweetened tea with lemon (temperature 60-70° F) is as refreshing as mineral water, and is also free of carbonation, which must be avoided during athletic activity. Apple juice is also an ideal drink for balancing mineral and fluid loss, while providing refreshment.

Tip: Don't allow yourself to be impressed by the promotional activities of producers of mineral drinks. The beverages consumed by pros on the sidelines of the playing field are not the same as the label on the bottle. Even great athletic stars frequently consume only mineral water from those containers during a competition.

An athlete of any level should never attempt to quench thirst during a competition with sugary or alcoholic drinks. Energy-intensive sports activities often draw heavily upon the detoxifying capacity of the liver — placing great stress on it. A far more agreeable and appropriate beverage after heavy exertion is non-carbonated bottled water, or a mixture of mineral water with fruit juice (e.g. apple juice). A refreshing glass of beer or other alcoholic beverages may be consumed a few hours later, after the body "cools down" and is at rest. Any type of alcoholic beverage consumed soon after competition places severe stress on the liver.

The evening before competition, one glass of beer or wine is allowed. These drinks contain valuable nutrients, vitamins, minerals, and trace elements. But, only one glass is allowed for athletes of adult age. In general, athletes are advised against alcoholic drinks, even if they are diluted. Large quantities of alcohol have a negative influence on the nervous system and coordination and often lead to damage of the stomach and mucous membranes, metabolic diseases, and high blood pressure.

Prohibition of Alcohol for Sports Injuries

After suffering an injury, any consumption of alcohol during the first 24 hours is strongly discouraged. Any level of alcohol will disturb the body's management of fluids as well as the healing process. The result: The injury will "draw water," that is to say, increased swelling may develop.

Conscious Nutrition

After a sports activity, a full meal should only be consumed when the body has calmed down a bit. You should eat — especially during breaks or half-time — something which is easily digested and rich in carbohydrates (such as bread products, rice, vegetables) to replenish diminished energy levels.

The meal just prior to training or competition should be consumed no later than three hours before — otherwise, the food will lie heavily in the stomach, when one has to perform at peak capacity within one to two hours. The meal should predominantly consist of easily digested carbohydrates (pasta, potatoes, rice), little fat!, protein and fiber, and not be too large. It is also wise to include a lightly spiced bouillon or tomato soup. A wholesome, well-rounded diet is not easy, especially for young athletes: A quick bite in the school cafeteria or local fast-food restaurant often becomes an inferior replacement for a balanced meal, which physical demands require.

The ideal athlete's diet is common in Southern Europe: the "Mediterranean Kitchen" with its pasta, vegetables, fish, fresh salads and foods marinated in olive oil. Olive oil is of special significance because it helps the distribution of saturated and unsaturated fatty acids; thus fat-soluble vitamins can be absorbed by the body. Italian soccer players usually register better laboratory results than their German and American colleagues, who frequently resort to poor nutrition. If there is a desire for meat, we recommend white meat, e.g. turkey or chicken, fish, lean cuts of pork, veal or even ostrich.

Meat Consumption

We know that meat is basic to tissue repair. It contains complete proteins. It also contains iron, zinc, and B-vitamins. Small portions of meat balanced with vegetables, noodles, potatoes, rice, and salads are the best options available to athletes.

Tip: The banana in sports: The feeling of hunger which arises during a long sports-match is frequently satisfied by eating a banana. The fruit is easily digested and well-tolerated by the system. The ripe banana contains up to 10% free glucose and 90% starch, which slowly splits into fructose and glucose. It also contains substances which quickly help to form saliva, thereby preventing "dry mouth". Finally, the banana contains a relatively large quantity of potassium — important for tissue cell regeneration. By contrast, an apple can lead to stomach upset because it contains large quantities of acid. Since competition has already caused an elevated adrenaline level, the stomach could be negatively affected by an increased acid burden.

Many world-class athletes prefer to eat a breakfast of hot cereal (an easily made meal: oatmeal cooked in water with a little salt). The advantages of this choice are many; it is highly nutritious, easy to digest, and flavorful. To improve the flavor, honey, cinnamon, or milk may be added.

AIDS

Practical tips for the preparation of diverse aids, such as "hot-ice," "ice-slurry," and healing packs.

About Ice Treatments: Just a few years ago, first aid with ice-spray and ice cubes was the last word. In recent years we have departed from it. The use of ice-cubes in a plastic bag is no longer considered the best form of therapy.

There are now improved alternatives for first aid to injured body parts, to keep the consequences of a violent impact from a blow, shove, kick, or fall, as minor as possible. Ask your pharmacist for recommended products.

"Hot-Ice" Treatment

"Hot-ice" is the ideal first aid remedy. The advantage of "hot-ice" is its ability to keep an injured area evenly cooled for hours without any cold damage. When one adds ice-cold water and a shot of rubbing alcohol, the ideal cooling temperature is reached (which lies slightly above 32° F). The circulation which nurtures the tissues is reduced, but not blocked. With plain ice, injured body parts often become over-chilled — the result is an over-reaction. When ice is removed, heat rushes into the chilled area. The blood vessels expand, and the circulation accelerates in order to equalize the temperature deficit in the affected body areas. As a consequence, the area one intended to cool actually becomes overheated.

How "Hot-Ice" is Produced: Place 2 quarts of water in a 5-quart tub or bucket and add about 30 ice cubes (alternatively, use a large bowl.) To keep the mixture cool, add additional ice cubes as necessary throughout the treatment. The optimal "hot-ice" temperature of 34º F is reached when the ice cubes have melted. Then, place two Ace bandages, one 3-1/2 inches wide and the other at least 4 inches wide, and a sponge, into the container filled with "hot-ice."

> **Tip:** Coaches and trainers should always have ice cubes available in the refrigerator or freezer-chest for ready use in case of injuries.

"Hot-Ice" Bandage: Wrap an Ace bandage (saturated with ice water) loosely and neatly around the injury. If pressure is indicated, place a cold, wet sponge on the affected area and proceed to wind the Ace bandage tightly around it. As a rule, the first "hot-ice" bandage should be left in place for 20 minutes, with additional applications as needed.

A pressure bandage must be removed for 4-5 minutes after the first 20-minute cooling. This helps the affected area to obtain necessary circulation. If the skin appears evenly red, a new bandage may be applied. For "hot-ice" bandages, the addition of arnica lotion (2 tbs in 1-2 quarts of water) has proven helpful. Pressure bandages should be re-applied 3-4 times after each pause of 4-5 minutes.

Ice-Spray

Ice-spray is still in use. However, we recommend its use only if the patient is wet from "hot-ice". In this case, the ice-spray does not form a crust, but remains damp and cool for a long time at the desired temperature (near 32° F). Never aim the ice-spray directly at dry skin. Use it only for injuries on small areas, such as fingers, shins, knees, or knuckles. Never spray on open wounds!

Caution: Be cautious with ice-spray and ice cubes, which are applied directly to the skin! Cold water makes much more sense. No harm can come from a bucket of water, but it may from ice. Ice, if used, should be placed as ice-slurry in a fabric (such as a stocking or sock) and be allowed to remain on the injured area no longer than 10 minutes, at most.

Cold water effects a slow but lasting contraction of the blood vessels and it reduces the spreading of pain and swelling. At the same time healing processes are able to continue, and there are no undesirable side effects (such as overheating) as with the reaction that occurs after treatment with ice.

Ice Water Pack

As an alternative to "hot-ice", a cold pack can also be applied. It is a two-part package that becomes activated when one pops the package with the hand or foot. The cold temperature is produced in the area of 32°-38° F through a chemical reaction.

The disadvantage compared to "hot-ice": A cold pack quickly loses its cold temperature and adapts to one's body heat, so that there is insufficient ongoing cooling. Advantages of the cold pack include easy handling and easy transport.

Ice Slurry/Ice Slush

Ice slurry is applied to bruises, strained muscles, knee ligaments injuries, and foot injuries.

Fill a clean knee-high stocking with crushed ice. This easily malleable mass is then placed on a hand towel and applied to body curves in the injured area. Fasten the ice to the affected area with an Ace bandage so that it remains in position.

Note: Ice slurry must not be placed directly on the skin, but wrapped in a wet hand towel.

Ice-Towels for Heat Regulation

As a heat-regulation device during extreme summer temperatures, we recommend that several towels (regular size) be placed in a vessel (such as a bucket or tub) along with ice water and prepared before breaks or half-time. The athletes should then regularly cool their legs and necks with iced towels. This prevents overheated bodies and sunstroke by reducing body temperature. Important note on hot days: Do not consume ice-cold drinks.

Rubbing Alcohol/ Witch Hazel Compress

Good old home remedies generally used for cooling purposes in the past are still available at the drugstore, and continue to be very effective. When needed (such as for a bruise), mix cold water with rubbing alcohol in a 1:5 proportion. Submerge a washcloth or hand towel in this solution and place it on the injury for 15-20 minutes, periodically adding more solution. The cooling effect is increased through the quick evaporation of the alcohol. Witch hazel has a similar effect.

Packs

Healing Earth Packs: Prepare packs such as Luvos Healing Earth packs (obtainable at health food stores) with a corresponding amount of arnica lotion or cream (in a proportion of 2 Tbs. arnica to 1 quart cold water). After cooling the mix in the refrigerator for about 3 hours, the Healing Earth mix is spread on the injured area thickly and evenly, and wrapped with a damp towel. Ideally, the pack should be left on overnight.

Fire Pack: Apply for pain in the back and neck, or stiff shoulders. Spread Flexall on the painful area with a tongue depressor. Then apply the following in sequence: Bath towel, plastic wrap, hot water bottle, or heating pad. This packing should be applied for 15-20 minutes, twice daily.

Important: If the skin cannot tolerate the increased heat this pack will generate, remove the hot pack or heating pad. In case of a stiff shoulder, rub the painful area uniformly with ice or a "water popsicle".

Tip: To make a "water popsicle": Fill a yogurt container or a small dixie cup with water. Place a small wooden popsicle stick into the cup and freeze it. Later, you can rub the ice-on-a-stick onto the painful area.

Medications

Our recommendation of certain medications and their dosages, and the references to diversified help and support, has been based on years of experience in our practice. One can also apply other medications of identical action or effect, depending on the decision of your physician.

Pain Pills: The intake of strong pain pills (narcotics) is advised only for emergency cases involving excruciating pain. They must be prescribed by a doctor. After taking analgesics, the pain is no longer felt. As a consequence, the injury (such as the laceration of a muscular fiber) frequently fails to get the necessary attention and the healing process is delayed.

WARMING UP / WARM-UP STRETCHES

Nobody loves it, but it should become the athlete's duty to stretch and loosen the muscles. These exercises are an integral component of the warm-up program for every athlete, whether part-time athlete or professional. Only a thorough warm-up (exercises) and warm-up-stretching (stationary exercises) attune the body to upcoming stress, raise it to performance-level temperature, improve skill and flexibility, and facilitate optimal performance.

The warm-up serves to produce a mild sweat while elevating the temperature of the body to performance level. It also promotes a harmonious collaboration between joint and muscle functions.

The athlete should expect to spend between 10-15 minutes for initial warm-up, with subsequent warm-up-stretching of around 4-5 minutes. This is a relatively small amount of time, and it is worthwhile in various ways for, like an automobile motor, the human body is capable of its best performance only after a few attempts have been made to warm it up and prepare it for moving. Through warm-ups and stretching, energy and adrenaline is released throughout the body and the risk of injury is lowered. Well-stretched ligaments and joints are ready for subsequent training or competition.

Therefore, we repeat our appeal to the athlete: Even if it is boring and seems difficult in the beginning, warming and warm-up-stretching should be part of the standard program before every training, start, or game. Good habits must be learned. Only the trainer or physical therapist can communicate the basic techniques which can later be done independently. When the athlete can appreciate the effect these exercises have on the body and is able to perform them routinely, it should be a habit.

Note: Warming-up should be specific, depending on the type of sport. Every athlete needs to stretch only those muscles which will later be used.

The athletic ability of a human being essentially depends on inherited qualities. The decisive factor of an ability depends on tissue structure and frame. Therefore, take heart! Do not compare your performance to that of another athlete.

Note: Children and youths who are still growing should not, and need not, learn these exercises.

Basic Rules for Warm-Up and Warm-Up-Stretching

The term warm-up is synonymous with a gentle exercise program that has nothing to do with old-fashioned rigid gymnastics and their choppy motions. It should be learned under proper guidance and practiced with patience in the beginning.

During stretching, force is not necessary. Forceful stretching and bad technique can lead to the risk of injury.

The muscles must not be stretched too often and for too long; otherwise the innate tension needed for competition is diminished or lost. A muscle cannot reach its optimal strength when it has been stretched beyond its relaxed capacity before the competition.

Here is how to do it right:

Increase your circulation with a 10-15 minute jog or endurance run and work-out (rotate the trunk, arms, legs, feet and hands).

With the development of a mild sweat, the time has come for the next step: 4-5 minutes warm-up stretching, stationary stretching exercises.

Stretch each of the individual muscles for 20 seconds until tension is felt. There should be a tugging sensation in the stretched muscle, but it must not hurt — especially in the joints.

Tip: During the warm-up program, the choice of clothing depends on the weather and is specific for the type of sport. So, the final phase of warming-up for soccer players is the uniform choice. By contrast, "track-and-fielders" are advised to shed their training outfit shortly before beginning competition — they must enter the race in "steaming" condition.

In order for the body to regenerate faster, an active and passive cool-down session must take place immediately after training or competition.

REGENERATION / "COOL DOWN"

The event is over; the goal has been reached; the game is concluded. Yet, for the athlete, the challenge is not finished. To restore performance capacity in maximum time, the "cool down" must be performed as soon as possible; that is, measures for active and passive regeneration must be carried out. True rest comes with the elimination of toxins as quickly as possible, thereby assisting the body to develop a rapid recuperation. A wait of even one day is too long. It makes it more difficult to obtain the proper benefits.

One must differentiate between active and passive regeneration. A passive measure cannot replace one that is active. For example, the ideal form of active regeneration for most athletes is a slow jog at the end of a sports event for 10-15 minutes, as is customary for "track-and-fielders". For soccer and tennis, this is not an option, because of security considerations and crowds. Alternatively, the locker room facilitates active regeneration by providing other methods of "cooling down," such as swimming, stretching and light exercises.

- Also recommended: 20 minutes on a stationary bicycle without extensive muscle exertion.
- After active exercises come passive ones. A generous shower with an increasingly warm temperature or, if possible, swimming for 10 minutes in warm water at 85-90º F, without work-out.
- If there is no possibility of a relaxing bath immediately following the event, one can obtain similar results one or two hours later in the bathtub at home. Positive effects become more pronounced from adding a handful of coarse salt to the warm water.
- Following a bath or swim, a brief sauna is very

beneficial. Wrap the body in a large towel or bathrobe and let it perspire. As an alternative try 10 minutes of stretching exercises or light exercises.

- A series of saunas (at most, two) are recommended only with reduced temperature: with mild perspiration developing over 6-8 minutes at approximately 140° F.
- Subsequently, one may consider a massage.
- After that, rest is in order.

Warm-Up Exercises/Stretching

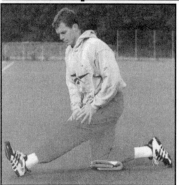

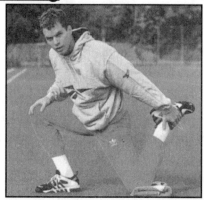

**UPPER THIGH /
BACK STRETCH:**
*The leg to be stretched is
placed forward, with knee
straight. The hands are
placed on the upper thigh
while pressing down until
the knee-joint is stretched.
The upper body bends
slightly forward at the hips,
with the eyes directed at the
toes. Duration: about 20
seconds.*

UPPER THIGH / VENTRAL STRETCH:
*Place the knee on the ground,
using a towel as padding. The
upper body is then thrust forward
above the bent knee. Hold the
ankle and pull the lower leg up
toward the buttocks. Duration:
about 20 seconds.*

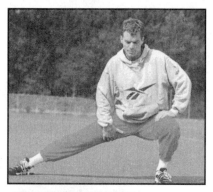

**UPPER THIGH /
OUTSIDE STRETCH:**
*The leg to be
stretched is posi-
tioned behind the
other leg. With
hands on the hips,
turn the upper
body in the
opposite direction.
Duration: about
20 seconds.*

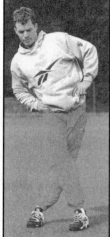

ADDUCTOR STRETCH:
*Position the leg alongside the
body and stretch it the full
length. The body's weight is
placed upon the bent leg, while
leaning slightly forward. The
buttocks are lowered and the
hand grabs the inside thigh of
the stretched leg. Duration:
about 20 seconds.*

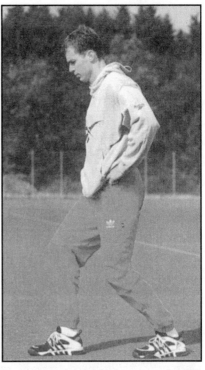

CALF STRETCH:
The leg to be stretched is positioned one step back. The heel is firmly pressed into the ground and the knee moves forward. Place the hands on the waist for support. Duration: about 20 seconds.

STRETCHING THE CALF MUSCLES:
Place both hands on the ground, keeping the body raised and the arms straight. The leg is stretched out with the knee straight and the foot flat on the ground. The other leg is bent with the toes of the foot hugging the Achilles tendon. The upper body leans forward. Duration: about 20 seconds.

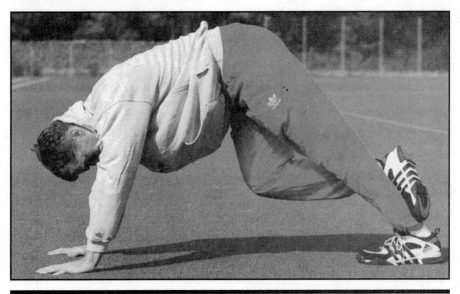

GLUTEAL (BUTTOCK) STRETCH:
Exercise 1: The athlete lies on his back. The leg to be stretched is bent at the knee and placed on the lower thigh of the other leg. The hands grasp 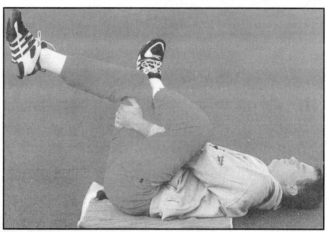 *the back of the lower thigh and pull it toward the chest. Duration: about 20 seconds.*

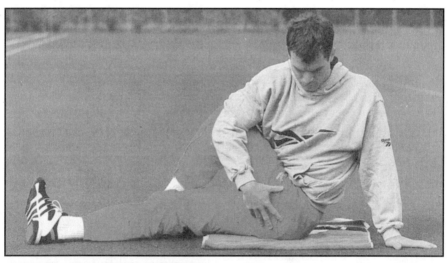

GLUTEAL (BUTTOCK) STRETCH:
Exercise 2: The athlete begins in a sitting position. Place the leg to be stretched at a right angle across the other leg. Hold this position. The hand clasps the upper thigh from the outside and the body is turned toward it. Elbow and hand draw the upper thigh and the knee inward. Duration: about 20 seconds.

BACK STRETCH:
Start the exercise while lying on the back. Clasp both knees and pull them toward the head. The head is pressed between the knees and held there. Duration: about 20 seconds.

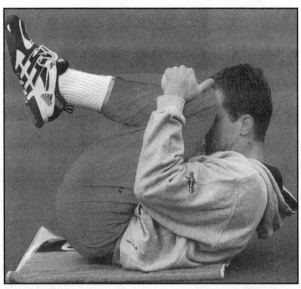

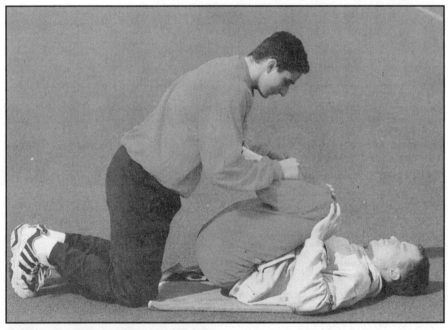

BACK STRETCH WITH PARTNER:
The reclining partner's back gets well stretched through the extreme pressure of both his feet on the chest of the kneeling partner. Duration: about 20 seconds

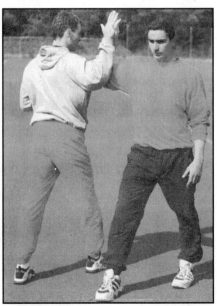

**CHEST STRETCH
WITH PARTNER:**
The partners stand facing each other. Each takes a half-step to the side, then raise right arms; join palms and elbows together. Each partner presses where palms and elbows join, moving forward slightly. Repeat the stretch on the left side. Duration: about 20 seconds.

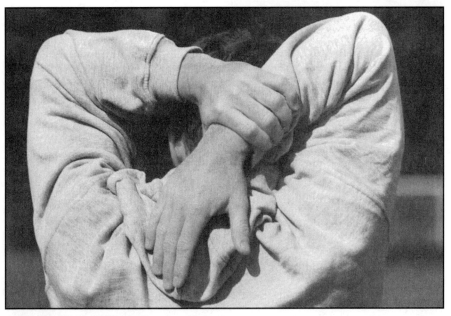

UPPER ARM STRETCH:
The upper wrist is clasped with the opposite hand and moved behind the head in the direction of the opposite shoulder blade. Duration: about 20 seconds.

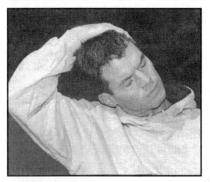

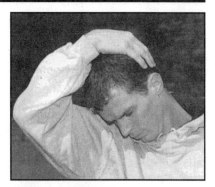

NECK STRETCH:
The head is bent slightly to the side and clasped by one hand. The shoulder and the arm of the opposite side are held downward so that a pulling sensation in the neck muscles occurs. Duration: about 20 seconds.

NECK STRETCH:
The head is slightly bent to the side and clasped by one hand; the head is then rotated. Duration: about 20 seconds.

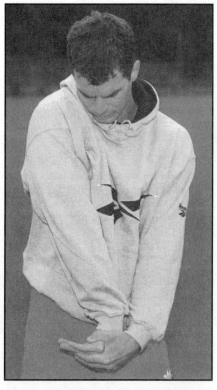

LOWER ARM STRETCH / EXTENSOR SIDE:
The arm to be stretched is held straight down; the hand is bent outward and clasped by the other hand which presses upward. Duration: about 20 seconds.

NOTES

Hastings House Book Publishers
Tel: 203-838-4083
Fax: 203-838-4084

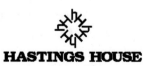

HASTINGS HOUSE

Functional Bandages

By "functional taping technique" or "taping" we use a series of practices that have proven themselves for many years and have been tested in many arenas. They are a method of medical care for prevention and therapy of injuries, disease, and changes in mobility systems. Taping techniques originate from functional anatomy and are predominantly accomplished with adhesives, elastic and/or non-elastic bandages.

Here are important points for avoiding mistakes in the application of tape bandages, especially when applying non-elastic tape.

Apply the tape in the following sequence:

1. Measuring: Unroll a length of tape which is appropriate for the planned application. Hold the tape roll loosely in the hand, avoiding any pressure of the thumb on the roll.
2. Application: Hold the tape taut. Select a suitable starting location on the body. For example, begin on the sole of the foot for a U-support at the ankle joint. Determine the precise length needed on the body.
3. Tear off: Do not tear the tape directly on the bandage; tear or cut before placing it.
4. Placement: Place the tape according to the planned procedure. While doing this, do not force the body into an unnatural position.
5. Shaping: With light pressure, shape the tape according to the body's contours. By wrapping in this manner, you will achieve a strong bond with the skin or the underlying bandage, as well as a secure fit.

> **Tip:** For better bonding of the tape to the skin, and easy removal of the bandage later, spray a tacky film on the skin beforehand. Ask your pharmacist for recommended products.

Note:
- The bandage enables healing; it must fit well.
- Wear comfortable clothing. When the foot or legs are bandaged wear comfortable, flat shoes.
- The importance and the chief advantage of taping lies in the high degree of mobility maintained. As long as it does not hurt, mobility accelerates the healing process.
- With arm and hand bandages, remove rings first. If swelling occurs, the rings can stop circulation and may have to be cut off. Mild swelling usually disappears when the limb is raised above the level of the heart.
- Protect tape bandages from dampness: It may make them tighter or cause them to lose their adhesive strength. An elastic bandage, or a stocking, loosely applied, will protect the area from getting soiled or damp.
- When taking a shower wear a plastic shower hat or post-operative wound cover (special shower protection is available at the drugstore) to protect the bandage.

Caution:
In case of the following complications, the bandage must be cut or removed immediately:
- Severe or increasing pain.
- Severe swelling, especially of the fingers and toes, which fails to be relieved by elevating the part.
- Blue or white discoloration of fingers or toes that does not decrease with elevating the limb above heart level.

- A feeling of numbness, tingling or itching (a feeling like ants running across the skin), or sudden limitation of movement.

> **Tip:** A strong itching sensation may indicate an inflammatory or allergic response by the skin. In this case the bandage must be replaced by a different one for sensitive skin.

Therapeutic Bandages

Therapeutic bandages should be applied soon after an injury. One should discontinue them as promptly as possible during the healing process. Otherwise, the body adapts to the support. This can lead to on-going problems in other parts of the body. For example, one could apply the bandages exclusively for competition, but gradually do without them for training.

Protective Bandages

As a precaution, therapeutic bandages should be applied for sports activities only on joints which are unstable or injured. Protective bandages are necessary for sports such as basketball, volleyball, handball, etc. which cause extreme stress to specific areas.

> **Tip:** As a rule, strechable cloth bandages should be used — not rubber bandages. Cloth bandages have a uniformly woven elasticity, but rubber bandages have rubber threads interwoven. Any bandages which double in length from a slight pull during their application are unsuitable. However, short, stretchable bandages (Ace bandages) are appropriate. Tape is used in supporting bandages for the ankle joints.

Ointment-Bandages

Here is the expert's way of applying an ointment-bandage: Spread the ointment thickly and evenly, preferably with a tongue depressor (or popsicle stick), on the affected area. Place a damp gauze compress on it and wrap it with an Ace bandage or other flexible-stretch bandage of an appropriate size.

You may also cut a piece of cotton or an absorbent compress to the desired size. Dampen it with water from a spray bottle, and spread the desired ointment on the pad with a tongue depressor. The ointment-compress is placed on the injury and then wrapped.

Important: An ointment-bandage must be damp before it is applied. If this is omitted, the compress dries up within a short time due to body heat and the ointment loses its effectiveness.

GUIDELINES FOR TAPING TECHNIQUE

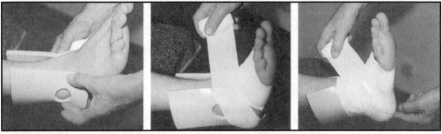

COMPRESSION BANDAGE WITH PRE-CUT FOAM RUBBER PADS AND AN ACE BANDAGE FOR AN ANKLE INJURY:
Submerge the foam pads in ice water, then place them on the inner and outer joints. Wrap them with an Ace bandage using medium pressure around the joint.

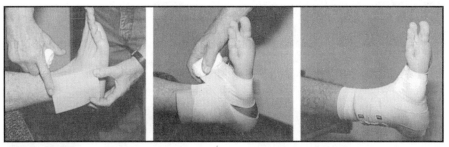

Alternative:
A pressure bandage using a sponge and Ace bandage for the ankle may be used. Submerge a sponge in ice water and place it on the injury. Then wrap it with a 3-inch wide Ace bandage, using medium pressure, with large overlapping to the middle of the lower calf.

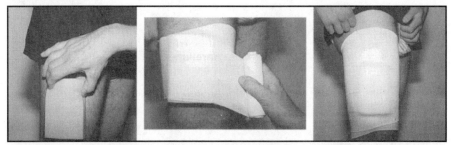

PRESSURE BANDAGE FOR A RUPTURED MUSCLE FIBER OR A MUSCLE CONTUSION OF THE UPPER THIGH:
Apply a sponge that has been submerged in ice water to the injured area with an Ace bandage about 4-5 inches wide, using strong pressure.

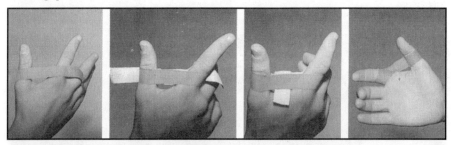

FOR AN INJURED THUMB (BASE JOINT OF THE THUMB) AFFIX THE THUMB TO THE INDEX FINGER:
A 3/4-inch wide taping strip connects the thumb and index finger at their base. At the center, the loop is fastened with a square strip.

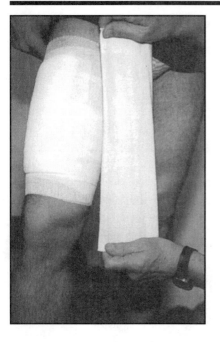
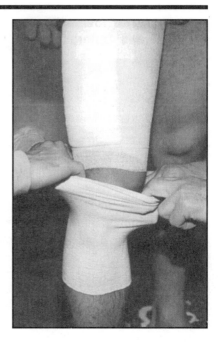

FOR A RUPTURED MUSCLE FIBER OR A MUSCLE CONTUSION OF THE UPPER THIGH:
Place a compress (folded gauze with cotton) which has been spread with ointment on the upper thigh. Bandage it with an adhesive wrapped in 3 or 4 layers. Finally, cover it with an elastic thigh brace.

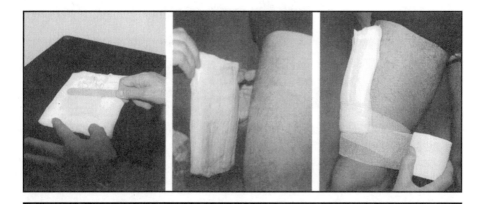

OINTMENT BANDAGE ON THE ANKLE BONE:

Spread ointment on a compress (folded gauze plus cotton) and place it on the injured area. Then fasten it with an adhesive bandage (or other large stretchy bandage) under moderate pressure. Fasten the ends with 2-3 strips of tape.

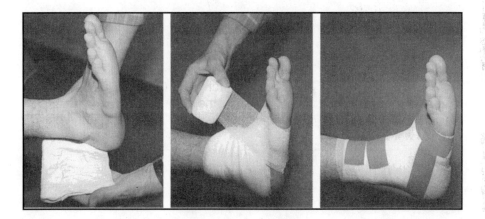

*UNDERLYING BANDAGE SECURED WITH
TAPE OR PRE-WRAP:*
*Wrap the foot with a bandage up to the
middle of the lower calf. Secure with 3
pieces of tape. Fasten the bandage at
the upper end near the calf using 2
pieces of tape. Then wrap the entire
casing, overlapping the tape to secure it
while using medium pressure.*

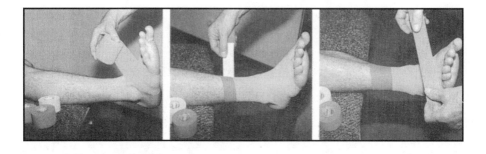

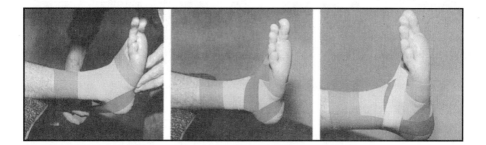

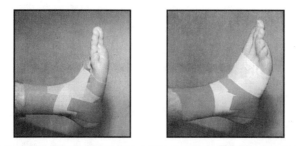

NOTES

All forms of Traumeel are available from:
Heel Inc.
1-800-621-7644

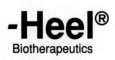

-**Heel**®
Biotherapeutics

NOTES

For more information about Marco Sport,
call Pro Nutrition at:
1-888-303-7668

First Aid Equipment

Fast and effective care for an injury through appropriate first aid frequently decides the later course of developments. The following provisions are recommended as a kit that is put together from supplies found in drugstores and sport specialty shops:

1. 6 Gauze compresses (3 pads 4 inches square, 3 pads 2 inches square)
2. 1 bottle of Disinfectant (peroxide, Bactine spray or tea tree oil)
3. 1 small box of Band-Aids
4. 1 adhesive bandage
5. 1 roll of 3-inch tape
6. 1 roll of one-inch tape
7. 1 roll tape, nonirritating or hypoallergenic
8. 2 Ace bandages (3 to 4 inches wide)
9. 1 blister bandage or moleskin
10. Instant ice pack
11. 1 cellulose sponge
12. 1 tube of antibiotic ointment (such as Betadine or triple anti-biotic ointment)
13. 1 bottle muscle relief ointment (Flexall, Cramergesic, Bengay or "Born Again")
14. 1 pair of scissors
15. 1 disposable razor
16. 2-3 Tongue depressors
17. A cooler for ice water

Important: After the use of supplies, replenish them!

NOTES

For more information about Wobenzym call:
1-888-4-VITAMINS
(1-888-484-8264)

Wobenzym®

WOBENZYM AND SPORTS INJURIES

The number of acute and delayed-onset injuries sustained during regular exercise and engagement in sports is not exactly known. With the increase in health consciousness, as more and more people exercise and increasingly participate in various sports, the number of athletic injuries is certainly on the rise. Roughly 80% of all athletic, or sports-related, injuries are lesions in the soft tissue, such as contusions and compressions. These lesions, and vascular ruptures attendant to them, cause swelling and pain.

SORE MUSCLES: Irrespective of the level of fitness from any form of physical exercise, if one begins to, say, jog, there will be sore muscles. Even if one becomes used to jogging on a regular basis, from time to time, muscles will become sore. There are three reasons for people to experience sore muscles:
1) Lack of Exercise;
2) Used to a Different Exercise; and
3) Increasing the Frequency and Intensity of Their Regular Exercise.

Soreness starts as a result of tiny tears (microtrauma) in the muscle, which is akin to a paper-cut on the finger. [It may be uncomfortable and may even be painful, but the finger remains functional.] With the onset of microtrauma, the body's defense mechanisms dispatch white blood cells to the rescue, and fluids move into spaces they normally do not occupy, resulting in swelling {Doenicke & Hoernecke, Deut. Z. Sportsmed.: 44, 214, 1993}. The swelling nudges nerve endings, causing soreness. It also stiffens the muscle, on occasion immobilizing it. Swelling and soreness often peak between 36 to 48 hours after the exercise regimen, which explains the appearance of soreness and muscle stiffness on the second day after exercise or playing sports.

There are two types of muscle soreness: Acute and delayed-onset muscle soreness (DOMS). Muscle soreness experienced during or immediately after exercise results, primarily, from the accumulation of waste products, such as hydrogen ions and lactic acid, and from fluid shift from the blood to the muscle. This fluid shift is the "muscle pump" that is discerned as discomfort or pain following heavy endurance or strength training. This type of muscle soreness normally disappears of its own accord within a few minutes to several hours after the exercise period.

In contrast, muscle soreness experienced a day or two after the exercise regimen, DOMS has only now begun to be fully understood. The DOMS ensues as a result of the body's inflammatory response in the muscle after exercise, since the white blood cell count tends to increase after activity, which causes muscle soreness.

Another view that accounts for DOMS holds that eccentric muscle action is responsible for delayed muscle soreness. During eccentric muscle contractions, the muscle lengthens as it contracts. The lowering regime in weight lifting, e.g., is an eccentric action. Also, running downhill causes the muscle to contract eccentrically {MacIntyre et al, APStracts: 2, 0486A, 1995}. It is worth noting that the muscle experiences greater damage and, hence, greater pain during eccentric contractions than during concentric contraction (i.e., when a muscle shortens during a contraction).

What happens during the 24 to 48 hour period before the onset of delayed muscle soreness? During this period, the repair process does not start immediately. As a result, the damage is further aggravated as calcium ions accumulate inside the muscle cells, leading to partial breakdown and rebuilding of the muscle cells. Further, the levels of chemicals such as bradykinin and histamines [the compounds that cause inflammation] increase, activating the nerve endings and a dull, diffuse sensation of pain is registered.

The muscles, however, do adapt! With persistent physical conditioning, the likelihood of damage is reduced, as the muscles become more resilient. Nonetheless, injuries do occur. In such cases, cooling, compression and cessation of physical activity may be called for. To mitigate the pain, a variety of topical and oral remedies are used. Some of these remedies have no significant side effects. It is possible, however, to hasten the recovery period and even to prevent such injuries from occurring by using natural enzyme combinations {Woerschhauser, S, Allgemeinemedizin: 19, 173, 1990}.

WHAT ARE ENZYMES? Enzymes are long chains interlinked of amino acids, the building blocks of life, and carry out a wide range of vital reactions in the body {Lopez et al., "Enzymes: The Fountain of Life," The Neville Press, Charleston, South Carolina, 1994}. Wobenzym is the best known oral enzyme formulation that has been shown to be effective in management of sports injuries {Kleine, M.-W., Deut. Z, Sportmedizin: 41, 126, 1990}. Wobenzym contains trypsin, chymotrypsin, pancreatine, papain, bromelain and the flavanoid, rutin.

HOW DO ENZYMES WORK? A cascade of reactions occurs after the body has sustained an injury. The intensity of these reactions, of course, depends upon the severity of the trauma. This implies that the sooner this cascade of reaction is interfered with, the more rapid would the convalescence be.

APPENDIX

Enzymes, after forming a complex with a_2-macroglobulin, migrate to the locale of injury. Diverse repair mechanisms commence to form a fibrin "sheath" around the traumatized site as microthrombi. As a result, the blood vessels are partially or completely blocked, and they become increasingly permeable. Consequently, the injury site is practically "decoupled" from normal blood circulation {Stauder et al., Natur- & Ganzheitmed.; 1, 68, 1988; Streiehhan, P., Verdauungskrankheiten: 7, 28, 1989; Streichhan et al., Der prak. Arzt: 14, 16, 1989}. Enzymes practically breach through the blood vessels and, as such, facilitate expeditious restoration of the normal environment at the injury site that, in turn, generates conditions in order for edema and hematoma to be quickly and efficiently resolved. As the recuperation process proceeds, development of further edema is inhibited by rutin that reduces the permeability of the blood vessels. This also helps mitigate pain sensation. It should be noted here that other pain-reducing remedies, such as nonsteroidal anti-inflammatory agents, do not reduce the levels of inflammation; rather they are known to support and accelerate the inflammatory response. In contrast, by working with the repair mechanisms of the body, systemic enzymes normalize inflammation and shorten the period of time to fully recover and, in fact, prevent any further injuries {Stauder et al., op.cit.}.

The enzyme *gemisch* rapidly becomes effective. Thus, in animal experiments, it was established that systemic enzymes have a beneficial effect as quickly as within 30 minutes after dispensation of Wobenzym {Kleine & Pabst, as cited in Kleine, op.cit.}.

In short, oral enzymes provide a superior corrective modality to manage athletic injuries of all sorts, from hematomas to distortion to post-operative convalescence.

October 6, 1998
Aftab J. Ahmed, Ph.D.
Director
R&D and Business Development
Marlyn Nutraceuticals/Naturally Vitamins
Scottsdale, Arizona